Celiac Mom

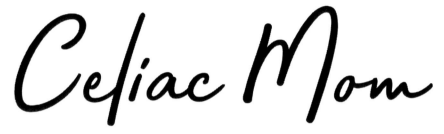

Celiac Mom

One family's gluten-free journey
after a daughter's diagnosis

ANN CAMPANELLA

The Bridge
Huntersville, NC

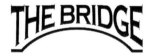

THE BRIDGE

Author's Note

This is a work of creative nonfiction. I have constructed the history of
my daughter's diagnosis and our family's journey into a gluten-free
lifestyle as accurately as possible using my own journals, medical
reports and discussions about events with my family and others who
were involved. Names of certain people, medical professionals,
organizations and businesses were changed to protect their privacy.
Any information about celiac disease and a healthy lifestyle is intended
for educational purposes only and should not be substituted for medical
advice from a doctor or healthcare provider.

ISBN-13: 978-0-578-70828-7

Produced in the United States of America

The Bridge
Huntersville, NC
www.TheBridgeBooks.com

For Sydney

*and all those
who have to say
goodbye to gluten*

Table of Contents

Prologue

A few hours still before dawn. My husband and I get up and shower, force ourselves to eat a small breakfast. I gather Sydney, still warm from sleep, into my arms and whisper, "It's time for us to go." She nods sleepily against me, her pale cheeks slightly damp.

I kiss the top of her head as I settle our five-year-old into her car seat. Are we doing the right thing? Will she be okay? Am I an overly concerned mom, putting my daughter through needless procedures? Have I blown her symptoms out of proportion in my imagination: her stomach pain, constipation, inability to nap, her small stature? Maybe all these things are normal, part of raising a healthy child.

This morning, the nurse at the hospital will prep her, and Sydney will be anesthetized. The doctor will take samples of the tissue in her small intestine, send it to a lab, and with any luck, within a few days, we will know whether or not our daughter has celiac disease.

I have never been a cook. In fact, Joel and I survived for years on a diet of microwave dinners and takeout food. Most weekends, we treated ourselves with a delicious four-inch high, wheat-bread sandwich made from our local chain whose name had the word "Bread" in it, topping off the meal with a huge chocolate chip cookie made with wheat flour.

A few hours later, we'd pick up subs (with whole wheat rolls, if we were being virtuous) or visit our favorite Italian restaurant for plates of baked ziti—noodles made with what else but wheat.

Wheat was our family's mainstay. We survived on it, planned around it, looked forward to it, even drooled over it. Gluten was a foreign concept. One of those weird words that overly health-conscious people used, people who liked to make others—like us—feel guilty.

All that would change when we learned that our daughter had celiac disease. What does it mean when someone is diagnosed with celiac? In medical terms, according to the Celiac Disease Foundation, when someone who has celiac eats gluten, an immune response is set off which damages the villi (tiny fingerlike projections) in the small intestine. When these villi are blunted, they can no longer absorb nutrients. This leads to autoimmune disorders and other health issues which can be serious such as anemia, arthritis, liver disorders, delayed growth and failure to thrive, to name a few.[1]

In human terms, my daughter was not being nourished. After breakfast, she'd rest on the couch holding her stomach. Her low energy kept her sitting still and playing with blocks and puzzles, instead of constantly being on the go like other toddlers. An intense heat in Sydney's body made her kick off her shoes and peel back her blankets, even in the dead of winter. She couldn't take long naps or sleep through the night—even through the age of five. And most concerning to me as her mother, she was not growing at a normal rate.

For our family, a celiac diagnosis meant that we had to accept a major change in our lives if we were going to support Sydney. Forevermore, I would become a detective on the lookout for any and all foods that contained gluten. It was one of those things that went beyond choice. It was a decision made for my husband and me, knit within our very DNA from the moment we met our daughter in the flesh, before she was born even. She was a precious, new part of our family, a miraculous gift from God. Of course, I would do this and much more. Anything it took to care for her, to keep her healthy, to help her thrive. This was a medical necessity for Sydney. The presence of gluten in her diet was damaging her intestines and keeping her malnourished.

From a practical standpoint, our small family suddenly found itself outside the norm. And it was my job as the mother to help us navigate this transition. We had to remove ourselves from the countless typical routines that involved food. I had to approach each meal with a new set of eyes, an awareness that a poison could be lurking, a food that could undermine my daughter's health was always close by. I had to figure out how to deconstruct our patterns around the grain my husband and I had spent a lifetime eating and find a way to build new habits and traditions that would not compromise Sydney's health—and ultimately ours—but instead provide nourishment.

For me, this diagnosis meant spending hours researching on the internet, cleaning out our pantry, setting up boundaries in my mind—not boundaries of resistance and craving, but boundaries that would hopefully bring life and health, energy and growth.

For months, even years, before we knew what was going on, I had spent evenings going over in my mind what Sydney had eaten; I had late-night discussions and arguments over "treats" my husband had slipped her. My mother's intuition told me that something was not right—horribly wrong, in fact. So, I monitored everything she ate, noted every reaction. I could tell that she felt better when she ate fruits and vegetables, that she became bloated after eating cookies and sugary foods, so I naturally limited those things.

I took Sydney to countless doctors and voiced my concerns over her stomach pains and chronic constipation. "Give her more fiber," I was told. "Make sure she's drinking enough."

When I pointed out that my daughter's height and weight didn't even register on the growth chart, I heard, "You worry too much." One doctor told me, "You and your husband are short." Joel is 5'7", shorter than average for a man, but I am 5'6½", which is taller than average for a woman. I was labeled a "nervous mom," and my concerns were dismissed. A digestive illness was never considered because Sydney didn't display the typical signs for celiac, which were constant diarrhea or vomiting.

I spent hours on the internet plugging her symptoms into search engines: severe constipation, delayed growth, sleeplessness, stomach pain, etc. On occasion, over time, certain words like "gluten" and "celiac" showed up amidst a constellation of other health concerns. But it was enough that when a specialist finally told me he wanted to run further tests and perform an endoscopy on Sydney because he suspected celiac, all the disparate pieces of my daughter's digestive issues and childhood history fluttered around me and finally began to fall into place. It was my first sign of hope.

My History

As a writer and a poet, I was never concerned about food. I didn't have the time or the inclination to think about cooking. My focus was on creating savory sentences and delectable metaphors, not meals. My mother, who had also been a writer, passed down to me her disinterest in all things culinary, so not spending time in the kitchen was normal for me.

Looking back, I realize that a good part of my life was spent in conflict with food. As a kid, I didn't think much about what I ate, as long as it was sweet. I remember holidays where I started the morning by nibbling the ears off my chocolate bunny and finished the day slightly sick to my stomach because I was full of jelly beans and crème-filled eggs. Not a carrot, green bean or even a slightly nutritious food passed my lips. My mother prepared her tasty, but uninspired, meals every night—spaghetti, meat loaf, tuna casserole—and somehow, as the youngest child in a family of six, I flew under the radar enough to exist mostly on a little bit of meat, some noodles, bread or crackers and a lot of candy.

I became aware of my relationship with food when I was a teenager and my family moved from the Panama Canal Zone to the coast of North Carolina. We had to leave my horses behind. Prior to that time, I had spent six days a week riding, running and playing hard. My body was long and lean, and I ate whatever I wanted.

After the move, I missed my horses and my old life terribly, and food became a comfort. I remember filling myself with Doritos and Red Hots, alternating between sweet and salty as I sat at the tiny kitchen table in our condo, wondering what I was going to do with my days now that I wasn't riding, and I didn't know anyone. I was still active— I took walks and ran on the beach almost every day. But forty-five minutes of exercise was nothing compared to my full days of nonstop activity in Panama.

In high school, I began to put on a few extra pounds. I hated the way my jeans were too tight, and the scale nudged up. Because of my tallish frame, I wasn't noticeably overweight, just perpetually uncomfortable in my body. At the same time, I was addicted to sugar. If I started the day off eating something sweet, I couldn't resist the siren call of more sweetness throughout the day.

My father called himself a "borderline diabetic." I didn't realize it at the time, but my body also reacted to sugar. Once it was in my system, my blood sugar must have risen to a level that kept me constantly craving something sweet. More often than not, my days were spent seeking my next sugar high.

It was only when I reached the age of fifty and stopped eating sugar completely that I finally felt free of a substance that had controlled me for most of my life. It was then that I finally began to understand how addictive my relationship with food and sweets had been.

Ten years earlier in 2001 when I was forty and pregnant with Sydney, I learned for the first time the importance of managing my blood sugar. I was tested for and diagnosed with gestational diabetes. Wanting to care for my baby (and being a wee bit obsessive), I took on the challenge of controlling my blood sugar while I was pregnant. I pricked my finger after every meal and tested my blood. By balancing protein and carbohydrates, I learned how to manage my cravings, for the most part. Sugar was still my favorite food group, so I would plan special small treats like a half cup of ice cream or a chocolate chip cookie on occasion, after I'd had some protein. I kept my blood sugar numbers within the diabetes guidelines but definitely noticed the spikes—not to mention the incessant desire to eat more—each time I ate something sweet.

I was so obsessed with sweetness that I froze a section of caramel cake baked by my best friend's mother for my husband and me to eat in the hospital after giving birth. After nine months of moderation, I couldn't wait to indulge again.

Little did I know that the "trauma" of giving birth probably prompted celiac to show itself in me. According to the Mayo Clinic, "Sometimes celiac disease is triggered—or becomes active for the first time—after surgery, pregnancy, childbirth, viral infection or severe emotional stress."[2] I say "probably" because my blood tests were inconclusive, and I have not had an endoscopy, which is considered the "gold standard" for diagnosing the disease.

After Sydney was born, I no longer restricted myself to a diabetic diet. I dropped any baby weight I'd been carrying without trying and, even while consuming additional calories, I had a hard time nourishing myself enough to be able to nurse Sydney. I indulged in pasta, cakes, cookies whenever it suited my fancy, and for the first time since being an active teenager, whatever I ate seemed to go right through me.

In actuality, I wasn't absorbing my food. My bowels were looser than normal. But, after a lifetime of semi-constipation, this didn't bother me. In fact, I thought maybe it was a good thing. My clothes fit easily, even—miracle of miracles—after having a baby. I didn't spend my time thinking or worrying about it though.

My focus was on Sydney, my beautiful daughter, over whom Joel and I were ecstatic. We had waited almost ten years for her, which had felt like a lifetime. I had undergone a series of miscarriages and cared for my mother who had Alzheimer's during that same period. It had been a desolate time of waiting, and before Sydney was born, we had begun to lose hope.

But suddenly our lives were filled with new light. We feasted on Sydney's milky white skin, her expressive, blueish-brown eyes, her curls of red hair, her perfectly shaped nose, her sweet lips. Everything about her was delectable. Mesmerizing. Everything, that is, except her crying, which would reach ear-piercing levels after dinner. Every night.

In the beginning, I breastfed her every few hours, determined to provide the best start for my little one. But no matter how much she nursed, or I pumped, I was only producing a few ounces of breast milk per feeding. It became clear that she needed more. So, I supplemented, trying various formulas after each one seemed to cause the same loud wailing.

Now, as I look back, although they manifested differently for each of us, I realize we were both showing signs of celiac.

New Mom, New Baby

*A*s a new mom, I had no idea what was normal for a baby. And I couldn't ask my own mother because of her Alzheimer's disease. So, I read and researched a lot!

During the first few months of euphoria, I accepted it as the norm to wake repeatedly throughout the night, sometimes just to peer at our cherubic girl. She slept in a crib in our room with her arms flung over her head, her eyelashes brushing her tiny cheeks like angel wings. It was heaven to bury my nose in her hair and inhale her sweet baby scent. This was what new moms did.

But as time went on, I was perplexed that Sydney's cries seemed louder and shriller, even after being nursed or receiving formula. Didn't babies fall asleep with a full stomach? Some evenings, when exhaustion took over, and knowing I'd have the graveyard shift, I'd ask Joel to walk her. But when her cries became piercing, I knew something wasn't right, and I'd take her back, holding her against me, letting her nurse just to soothe her. Often, I let her sleep with us. It was easier to make room for her in the bed than walk a few steps over to her crib multiple times a night in my zombie-like, sleep-deprived state.

Perhaps I perpetuated a routine where she learned that crying would bring comfort from Mama. That's a good thing, right? In those early months, I felt as if every cell in my body was programmed to do whatever it took to soothe my baby. The motherhood books I read

9

affirmed this thinking: "Never let a baby under six months cry it out." "Babies need comfort, not training." I took these words to heart and imagined that when Sydney was older, I could shift these habits and teach her to self soothe. Only that didn't happen.

As the days and weeks went on, there was teething and more crying. On a good night, Sydney woke up two or three times. On a bad one, she was up every hour.

Even when Sydney started eating solid food, nothing changed. If anything, her crying jags got worse. And, as usual, they were ear-piercing, the kind that made me feel as if a sharp knife was slicing into my chest. It was clear she was uncomfortable, maybe even in pain.

When I brought up my concern with the doctor, or other more experienced parents, they would smile indulgently. "All babies cry, Ann. Maybe she has a little colic. You'll get through it."

There was no easy time to make a transition and move Sydney into the nursery we'd prepared for her. In my sleep-deprived state, I joked with Joel: "This won't last forever. How many teenagers sleep with their parents?"

Toddlerhood

When Sydney became a toddler, her growth seemed to just stall out. The other moms I knew went through new clothes for their babies like water. Every time they turned around their child was in a new size.

Sydney had gained weight as a baby *very* slowly. I couldn't help but notice that the points on her growth chart were always near the bottom, that is, if her height and weight made the growth chart at all. I asked my doctor about this at each Well Baby Visit, but I was always reassured that everything was normal.

As a toddler, Sydney wore the same clothes for a few years. Granted, I usually purchased things on the slightly large side, and she grew attached to certain kitty shirts, so she didn't want to give them up, even when her belly button was showing. But I'm talking *years*!

How many kids wear the same Halloween costume three years in a row? Sydney's kitty costume started out a little roomy and eventually grew snug. But still…three *years*?!

It also became obvious to me that Sydney's growth wasn't normal when she began preschool. Her classmates were head and shoulders taller than her, and they kept stretching upwards in height, while Sydney's growth spurts were miniscule, measured in millimeters rather than centimeters or inches.

What was confusing was that her belly was round—bloated and inflamed, I later learned—making me wonder if she was overeating. Her behavior fanned my concerns.

We ate regular meals, and I tried to always have fresh fruit and other snacks available any time during the day. At dinner, no matter what I served, Sydney would ask for huge helpings and have no trouble putting away everything on her plate. As soon as the dishes were cleared, she would begin whining that she was hungry. Sometimes, within a few minutes of each other, she'd down two complete meals! I thought toddlers were supposed to be picky eaters. But mine sure wasn't.

Often, I'd look at her swollen belly, and shake my head. "No, Sweetie. It's not time to eat right now. You just had dinner." I thought I was being a good mom, teaching her limits. But to my horror, after her diagnosis of celiac, I realized that she had literally been starving! Her intestines were irritated, and her little body had not been able to absorb what she had eaten, so she was naturally hungry right after dinner. She could have eaten all day, and if her food contained gluten, as much of it did, not been able to satisfy herself. My heart aches now for what she must have been going through.

To Sleep or Not to Sleep

S leep deprivation is a typical issue for parents of babies—but for toddlers? As I look back, I realize our situation went way beyond normal. From the beginning, it had been a challenge to get Sydney to fall asleep. When she was a baby, we stumbled upon the method of putting her into her stroller and rolling it through the house. After forty-five minutes or an hour, she might begin to drift off. But if we stopped rolling too soon, or if I tried to move her, it was all for naught, and we'd have to start the whole process over—sometimes two or three times.

As a toddler, Sydney loved it when I read to her, so we had a routine each night. After Joel gave her a bath, I'd either sit on the floor with a stack of books beside me or hold her on my lap in the rocking chair. After each story, Sydney would turn to me and ask in the sweetest little voice, "One moa?" Of course, I always obliged. I kept expecting her to lean her head back and close her eyes, or at least begin yawning. But that never happened.

After reading a dozen or more books, I would put Sydney in her crib, rub her back and quietly step out of the room. Then the crying would begin. I tried all the tricks suggested by the parenting books: back away slowly, leave a nightlight on, play soft music, stand outside her room and come in after longer and longer intervals. Nothing worked.

Joel and I even tried letting Sydney "cry it out," but she would wail deep into the night, not falling asleep for hours. For Joel who had to get up and go to work in the morning and for me who had to stay awake and care for her the next day, it was untenable to listen to her cries as we counted down the hours of sleep we were missing. Not to mention my heart was breaking at the sound of her misery, and my nerves were on edge from the high-pitched sound of her crying. So, I usually broke down, somewhere into the second hour, scooped her up, covered her head with kisses and brought her up to bed with us. There she would sleep fitfully, only drifting off when her body was splayed out on top of mine.

Before dawn, Sydney was up and ready to play. Bleary-eyed, I tried to encourage her to stay asleep for a few more minutes. But she was bright-eyed and wide awake, full of smiles and ready to start her day.

After a morning of playing with blocks, building train tracks or going to the park to meet a friend, I'd feed Sydney and put her down for a nap. "Down for a nap" was just an expression in our house because actual sleep was rare. She would play with her stuffed animals, talking and singing to them for thirty minutes, occasionally forty-five minutes or an hour. I would go upstairs, crack my bedroom door and lie down to read and nap myself, listening to the spiral of her sweet voice repeating phrases from the day.

I often woke with a start to the sound of crying. It usually started as a whimper and gained force the longer I waited.

Part of me knew that jumping up and responding to Sydney's cries was only teaching her that it worked: if you cry, Mommy will appear. But without my own mother to give me gentle direction about what I was doing, I had no guidance other than the words of friends or parenting experts in books or newspaper columns. So, I had to rely on my own feelings and inexperienced judgment.

During this time of my life, I existed within a strange age continuum. I was exactly in the middle—forty years older than Sydney and forty years younger than my mom. My mother had been gradually slipping into Alzheimer's for years, and she seemed to be near the end of her life by the time Sydney was born. So, I spent my days holding onto the last threads of my mother as I was raising my young daughter who was full of light and the sweetness of new life.

Caring for my mother and Sydney at the same time left me in a state of heightened awareness. At times, when my mother had fallen or stopped eating, it felt as if each breath might be her last. Each moment seemed to stretch and fill with a sacred beauty, and I wanted to fully absorb and be present for my loved ones—all of them. I wanted to appreciate my time with Mom as well as bathe myself in the bright glow of my precious daughter and remind myself of the circle of life.

When Sydney cried, I felt it throughout my body; the sound coursed through my veins, and every part of me wanted to soothe her. It was as if we were still connected—two parts of a larger organism—and it soothed something deep inside me to hold her, stroke her damp hair and petal-soft skin. When she was at peace, my world was brighter.

I also sensed that, at least sometimes, Sydney's crying might be connected to a kind of physical pain, something different from the cries that came from being wet or hungry, tired or scared. When she felt good, Sydney was so full of joy; she had a sparkling effervescence that overflowed to everyone around her. Her smile lit up her face as laughter bubbled out of her. One of my friends said, "Sydney is the smile-iest child I've ever known."

But there were periods when something seemed to shadow that part of her. I didn't understand it at the time. But, in looking back, it's easy to see how her inflamed digestive tract became that shadow, a low-level irritant muting her joy.

I was in shock when I learned that one of Sydney's friends, who we often met at the park, would go home and sleep for two, sometimes three or more hours. Then she'd wake up and go back to bed in the evening by 8 p.m.

If Sydney happened to nap for twenty or thirty minutes (God forbid any longer!), it was impossible for her to go to sleep before 10 or 11 p.m. And even during the best of nights, when she fell asleep at the early hour of 9 p.m., she would wake up crying at least a couple of times during the night.

Sleep was a rare commodity for either of us during the toddler years. Somehow Joel had always been able to sleep, (even through Sydney's ear-piercing cries). But I often felt like the walking dead. At the time, I had no idea that any of this might be related to celiac disease.

It's hard to believe, but Sydney did not sleep through the night until she was five years old. This first full night of sleep came the day after her first day of eating gluten free.

How I wish I could have a redo for those years. If only I had known, I would have lavished Sydney with food. Gluten-free food. Food that would nourish her and not harm her. Food that would fill her belly and help her sleep. I wish I had known what was wrong. That we both could have slept. But I didn't know.

Fairhaven

*I*n the fall of 2002, around the time Sydney turned one, we moved my mother from an assisted living facility near the coast of North Carolina to a specialized Alzheimer's facility in the Charlotte area. Over the next few years, Mom's health gradually deteriorated, and we made the decision to move her to a local nursing home. When Sydney was four years old, my mother's condition worsened again. Mom had been living with Alzheimer's for over ten years, and my family had been sharing the caregiving during that time.

My mother had a series of falls that spring that were devastating to me. As far as we could tell, she must have leaned slightly forward in her wheelchair and didn't have the muscle tone or the awareness to pull her body back. So, she flopped over like a ragdoll, breaking the fall with her face. This happened twice within a couple of weeks. Each time she was rushed to the hospital, and I left Sydney in Joel's care as I met my mother in the emergency room. I held back tears and tried to smile encouragingly as bruises blossomed across her forehead and cheeks. Mom, utterly confused and hardly able to speak, looked out at me from swollen, blackening eyes.

Amazingly, my mother recovered from these falls, but the hospitalizations continued throughout the spring and summer for various reasons—she contracted a virus and couldn't keep food down, her blood sugar had skyrocketed, etc. Each visit to the hospital was stressful and exhausting. My siblings and I took shifts and sometimes stayed through the night. It was hard for me to catch up on my rest. Sydney wasn't sleeping well to begin with, and she probably picked up on my anxiety which caused her to wake more often than usual during this time of intense caretaking.

Late August of 2006, the month before Sydney turned five, I told Joel we needed to get away. I somehow had to break the cycle of worry over my mother and sleepless nights. Maybe getting away would improve Sydney's sleep too.

I wasn't sure how we could leave with Mom's health hanging in the balance, but I knew it was important. She had been teetering on the edge between life and death for months, and I needed a break, a time to relax and put my mind at rest.

The three of us hadn't been on vacation together, other than visiting our families, since Sydney was born. Joel relied on me to plan family getaways, and I simply hadn't had the energy to do it. Time away with just the three of us became a priority, and I knew it would be a balm for my physical and emotional weariness.

I mentioned in passing to my pastor that I was looking for a relaxing place where our family could enjoy being together for a couple of days, and he suggested Fairhaven Ministries. Just the name sounded soothing. When I looked it up on the internet, I saw a handful of chalets on a pristine mountain in Tennessee, less than three hours away. Fairhaven was created as a retreat center for people in ministry, and it was also open for laypeople. There were over a dozen chalets sprinkled around the hundred-acre property. Each one had a downstairs bedroom, a loft, a full deck with a nature view and a small kitchen. The property had a duck pond, trails that wound along a creek and a tiny, picturesque chapel. The main lodge housed a library and a gift shop that sold hand-made items and lent out board and lawn games. It looked perfect.

I contacted my brother and asked if he could be available to watch over Mom while we were away. He was willing and happy to be on call.

It was a joy to spend a few hours in the car, heading to someplace new. I could feel the stress from my caregiving role evaporating as we wound our way up into the mountains.

After checking in at Fairhaven's main lodge and scoping out the stash of games available to borrow, we drove past the pond where a small flock of ducks rested in the shade. Just beyond the water was the driveway to our chalet. It sat nestled on the mountain with its front windows and deck facing the valley.

The first thing I noticed as we opened the door was a jar of freshly baked chocolate chip cookies on the table—a treat we would all enjoy! We unpacked our bag of breakfast and lunch foods and settled in. During our three days and two nights, we quickly established a routine at our home away from home.

That afternoon, the duck pond was our first stop. The hosts provided a bag of stale bread (made from wheat) for guests to feed the ducks. Sydney stood on a rock that jutted into the water and threw crumbs into their open beaks.

In the morning, we ate breakfast then took a short hike, ending up at the pond again for more duck feeding. Sydney and the ducks fell in love. They could hear her coming.

"Here, duckies," she'd sing, as we walked toward the pond. The ducks paddled from the far bank where they'd been napping, a small flotilla heading straight for Sydney. She made sure to give each of them a similar amount of bread. If one got impatient, she'd scold him gently. "Wait your turn," she'd say, then she'd toss a rolled-up ball of bread over his head to make him swim in the opposite direction to make room for the smaller ducks.

She could have spent all day with them. But I reminded her that ducks napped after their meals, just like children. It never occurred to me to brush the crumbs from her hands.

After leaving the pond, we returned to the chalet to read and play games. I made sandwiches with whole wheat bread for lunch. Then, like the ducks, we napped—or rather Joel and I napped while Sydney played with her stuffed animals. Later, we took another hike around the property, played more games and made a trip into town for dinner and ice cream. The hardest thing about dinner was making sure we found a restaurant that served food that I liked. Being a picky eater, I'd check the menu before we sat down to be sure there was something I would enjoy eating.

Sleep wasn't magically restored. We were still eating gluten, and Sydney wasn't wild about sleeping in the loft, away from us, even with her menagerie of stuffed animals. At night, we tried various approaches—I did the usual routine (books, prayer time and a story about the ducks), read a few extra books, laid my head on the pillow with her and pretended to fall asleep, hoping she'd get tired. She did, but not enough to be comfortable sleeping on her own.

Eventually, I told her she could join us in our room. We made a bed out of blankets on the floor, and sometime during the night, she climbed in with us. Even if my sleep was interrupted, it was better than normal. I was able to take naps at Fairhaven. Knowing how exhausted I was, Joel would get up in the morning when he heard Sydney stirring and play a game with her, giving me an extra hour of sleep.

Our few days away at Fairhaven were a gift. To step away from my role as a caretaker for my mom and to be surrounded by nature on a quiet mountainside was good for my soul. I wasn't exactly looking forward to returning home, yet I felt more rested and fortified than I had in months.

Sydney burst into tears as we left Fairhaven and began driving down the mountain. "Who will feed the duckies?" she cried. "They need breakfast, lunch and dinner!" The only way I could console her was to promise that we'd send a loaf of bread to the hosts when we got home. She continued to cry intermittently, and she complained that her stomach hurt. She wiped her eyes and her mouth with hands that had the remnants of wheat crumbs on them. Little did we know that throwing bread to the ducks three times a day had likely made her symptoms worse.

Sugar Cookies

*O*ver Christmas that year, Sydney and I made sugar cookies. Even though I wasn't a cook, holiday baking held special memories for me. I remembered the days of old when I measured flour and sugar as my mother read aloud from the *Joy of Cooking.* Making Christmas cookies was what mothers and daughters did; it was a precious bonding experience. I could set aside my concerns over Sydney's diet and sugar intake for the day.

Dressed in black pants and her favorite black Halloween shirt with a gold kitty on the front, Sydney stood on a stool beside me and helped measure and stir the dry ingredients. I creamed the butter and sugar, and she poured the flour mixture into my bowl.

I thought nothing of the white cloud that hovered momentarily in the air. We sprinkled flour liberally between sheets of waxed paper, so we could roll the dough out easily and it wouldn't stick. Sydney's shirt had patches of white where she wiped her flour-caked hands. Even her face and hair sported white streaks. Flour had spilled on the counters and the floor.

I smiled as she nibbled at the edges of leftover dough. This was a tradition. The kitchen would need to be wiped down and so would she. But we were having fun in the process.

We decorated with icing, red and green sprinkles and chocolate chips. When our snowmen or stars broke in half, we giggled and ate them. So what if we hadn't had dinner first. This was Christmastime.

Sydney made a few trips to the bathroom, which (despite my carefree attitude) I couldn't help but notice. Maybe she had a touch of diarrhea from a virus. It was December and half the kids in her preschool had been sick.

In looking back, I realized this was the first time Sydney showed one of the more recognizable signs of celiac—diarrhea, which is typically caused by malabsorption. With so much gluten in the air and in her system, her body must have been overwhelmed and her system inflamed, the tiny villi lining her intestines were likely so blunted that nothing could be absorbed. This symptom was so rare for Sydney that I never mentioned it to our family doctor, which was probably one reason why she never suspected celiac.

The diarrhea disappeared after Christmas, and the constipation returned. I'm not sure why. But I suspect it had to do with the fact that Sydney wasn't getting enough food. Even eating two dinners back to back, she wasn't absorbing nutrients from these meals. So, her body may have been "holding on" to what normally would have been "passing through."

Sydney continued on with preschool. She was active and happy, always excited for the next activity or visitor. She was already reading and memorizing books that I read frequently to her. She loved to write, draw and act out stories. Her bright mind was always moving. But still she wasn't sleeping well, had frequent stomachaches and the skin under her eyes looked bruised. Something wasn't right.

A Glimpse of Hope

$\mathcal{A}$ few weeks later, after the holidays had passed, I was sitting next to my friend Jill at a basketball game. Joel and I had been season ticket holders for Davidson basketball since we'd moved back to the area nine years before Sydney's birth. Now, we often brought her to games with us.

Jill and I had been workout buddies at the Y long before Sydney was born, and we had been seatmates at Davidson games for years. She knew about my mother's Alzheimer's, and her mom eventually developed the disease too. So, we were used to talking about health issues.

Jill had watched Sydney grow from the days I sat her on my lap as a baby and cupped my hands over her ears to protect them from the loud buzzer that signaled the end of timeouts until now. Even though Sydney was five, with her tiny stature, she more closely resembled a three-year-old.

This particular evening, Jill and I arrived a few minutes before the game, and I shared with her my concerns about Sydney: her bloated belly, her stomach pain, her delayed growth. I told her I had been researching over the holidays, trying to understand what was behind these symptoms. Jill listened, focusing for a moment on the court where the basketball players were warming up. I could tell she had something she wanted to say, but perhaps wasn't sure how to do it.

She slowly began telling me about her college roommate's son. His dentist had pointed his parents toward the fact that he might have a growth disorder. "His family members were all small, so no one thought anything about it," she said. Jill looked me in the eye before continuing.

I nodded.

"They gave him growth hormones," she said. "He ended up being 'normal-sized.'"

"Growth hormones," I repeated, releasing a breath I'd been holding.

We had a brief conversation about how growth hormones worked and about the fact that they had to be administered before puberty ended. Puberty was still a long way off for Sydney, but if she ended up needing growth hormones, it wasn't too soon to begin looking into them. I took another deep breath.

Jill said the conversation she'd had with her college roommate got her thinking about her niece, Maggie. She had apparently been so small that her friends used to carry her around, way beyond the age when that might have been cute. Her niece was tested by an endocrinologist, and the doctor was eventually able to diagnose and treat her.

"Do you know the name of this doctor?" I asked.

She smiled. "I do. And he's right here in Charlotte."

I jotted down the doctor's name. Twin spirals of hope and anxiety rose inside me. Hope that we could finally understand what was behind Sydney's delayed growth and concern over what might be causing it.

That night after the game, I looked up growth hormones on the internet. I wasn't sure how I felt about them. The idea of giving them to Sydney was scary. There was a small window of time (before she finished puberty) when they would be effective. It would mean daily shots. And what about possible side effects?

I imagined the extremes: Sydney as a tiny adult, never growing beyond her prepubescent height...and then my daughter suddenly elongated into an unnaturally tall woman with stilt-like legs. I didn't care if she was short or tall. I loved Sydney for who she was, not her size. But, as her mother, I wanted to spare her the pain of being way outside the norm. My mind was spinning, and I knew I was getting ahead of myself. It was time to talk with Joel.

As we were getting ready for bed, I told my husband about the doctor Jill had recommended. And I quickly mentioned the possibility of growth hormones and how Jill's friend's son had been treated with them.

Over the past many months, I'd spent hours in late-night conversations with Joel, sharing my concerns and giving him evidence of Sydney's health issues. Part of me hoped to turn my husband into someone as vigilant as I was about Sydney's diet. That hadn't happened. But Joel still trusted my instincts regarding Sydney and the medical concerns I had for her. Either that, or he was tired of hearing me talk about the same thing over and over.

"Go ahead and contact him," he said.

Joel has an uncanny ability to cut through the tangle of my emotions and create a clear path for us to follow. But I needed to know if he was "all in" or just trying to pacify me.

I turned to face him. "Are you sure?"

"What do we have to lose?" he said. "If she's healthy, you'll feel better knowing, and if she's not, maybe he can help us."

"It won't be cheap," I said, almost adding, "But what's more valuable than our daughter's health?" A cliché statement, but like most clichés, it was true.

I watched Joel's reaction and realized I didn't need to say those words. My husband's face had turned solemn. His eyebrows lowered and any trace of lightheartedness left his voice as he spoke: "Do it."

Dr. V

*T*he next morning, I called Dr. V's office and made an appointment for Sydney. A few weeks later, Joel and I picked up our daughter from preschool and drove into Charlotte to meet the doctor. I would do the talking, but I felt it was important for Joel to be there to help him understand whatever it was we were facing and to have his support.

I had filled out extensive paperwork the week before, and Dr. V now asked me a series of questions about Sydney. Based on my answers, the doctor told me he had already narrowed down the possibilities.

He measured Sydney's height and gave us an estimate of how tall she would be as an adult based on her current growth rate: between 4'8" and 4'11". Even though these numbers confirmed my suspicions, it was distressing to hear that something was indeed affecting Sydney's growth. The doctor also gave us an order for an x-ray of Sydney's right hand. Based on measurements, he could conclude whether her bones were on track or behind their normal growth pattern. If they were behind, it meant something had slowed her growth, and she might be able to catch up if he could uncover the cause. This gave me hope.

Dr. V would need to draw some blood from Sydney and test her for a handful of health issues. Celiac was a definite possibility, but he wanted to rule out a few other things. They included various endocrine diseases which involved inadequate production of the thyroid hormone, which is necessary for bone growth. He also mentioned Turner's syndrome, a rare genetic disorder in girls who are missing an X chromosome.

Each condition the doctor described sent a tiny surge of adrenaline through my body. Another topic to research, another avenue to explore. Whatever we were up against, I wanted to be ready, to provide the best possible support and the most normal life for our precious daughter. The doctor patiently answered all my questions, and at the end, I hung my hope on the fact that he suspected celiac.

When Sydney heard the phrase "blood test," her eyes grew wide. Before coming to the doctor's office, she had asked me if she would have to have another "blood shot"—her made-up phrase combining "blood test" and "shot." I had been sketchy with her, not wanting to fan her fears. "We're just going to talk with the doctor today. I don't know what he's going to say. If he says you need a blood test, we'll do it. But only if it's absolutely necessary."

Thankfully, the nurse was quick and gentle with the needle. Joel and I promised Sydney a special treat afterwards. All we had to do now was wait.

A few days later, I got a call from Dr. V's office. They needed a few more blood tests.

"More?" I groaned. "But she's already been through this."

The nurse was apologetic. She wasn't sure where the mistake had been made, but the doctor needed more information to rule out certain conditions and make a correct diagnosis. She suggested I take Sydney to the lab at our regular doctor's office, so it wouldn't be so traumatic.

I sighed heavily. I hated for Sydney to have to have more blood drawn. But we were so close. It had to be done.

The next afternoon, I drove with Sydney over to the lab. She looked at me with big eyes and asked, "Is it going to hurt?"

"Maybe a little," I responded. I have always told her the truth, and she knows she can trust me. "Only for a second though. It will be over so fast."

How many five-year-olds could withstand a needle going into their arm and drawing out five or six vials of blood? She was tiny, head and shoulders smaller than all her preschool classmates. She didn't have that much blood to give. Yet, she was stoic.

In the lab, Sydney looked away as I had cautioned her so as not to see the needle. I held her on my lap and felt her tense up then relax as I reminded her, "Just breathe. It will be over soon."

I saw the tears swimming at the edges of her eyes. But she didn't let them spill until we stepped into the hall away from the nurses. She gripped my hand and pressed into me. I leaned down and gathered her small, warm body into my arms, and she quietly sobbed against my shoulder.

"You were so brave." I said, feeling the tears prick my own eyes. "So brave."

We had to wait for the next appointment to get the results of the blood test. According to Dr. V, the tTG/IgA tests used to measure antibodies produced by Sydney's immune system were inconclusive.

Her tTG (anti-tissue transglutaminase) count was 2, which was within normal range, and her IgA (immunoglobulin A) count was 23.9, which was considered borderline. I didn't fully understand what these letters and numbers meant, but the word "borderline" raised another flag in my mind.

Dr. V also studied the grey and white x-ray we'd had done of Sydney's right hand. He measured the length of her bones and concluded that they were a year and a half behind where they should be at her current age of five.

"That's good," he said. "It means that if we can treat whatever has slowed her growth, she should be able to catch up."

Based on Sydney's symptoms and the doctor's experience, he told us there was a good chance our daughter had celiac disease. He recommended that she have an endoscopy, the results of which would likely confirm or deny his suspicions.

I felt giddy with relief and the hope that an actual diagnosis might be within our grasp. All of my concerns, my late-night internet surfing, my awareness that something had been wrong with Sydney's digestion might be founded. It was the first time I had a doctor's confirmation that I could actually be on the right path.

Dr. V had his staff set up an appointment for us with Dr. S, a pediatric gastroenterologist who would perform the endoscopy on Sydney. We would see this new doctor in two weeks.

Two-Week Trial

S ince there seemed to be a good chance that Sydney had celiac disease, I thought we might as well get a head start on things. I made the effort to clear anything that contained gluten from Sydney's diet.

Gluten was clearly the devil. From my reading, I knew that it was found in grains such as wheat, barley and rye, and that it was the sticky stuff that held bread together. In the digestive tract of someone with celiac, it caused an inflammatory response because the immune system reacted to gluten as if it were an invader, attacking both the intestinal wall and the gluten. If Sydney had celiac, it meant that anything containing gluten—bread, cakes, cookies, pasta, etc.—would cause damage to her gut. It was overwhelming to think about.

But I had to stay in the moment. This was just a two-week trial. Surely, I could find enough gluten-free food to feed a five-year-old for fourteen days. And if not, it wouldn't be the end of the world if a little wheat slipped back in. After all, a little bit of gluten had to be better than a lot of gluten, I reasoned. Besides, we would know more soon. Maybe this trial would all be for naught. For now, removing gluten (or attempting to remove it) from Sydney's diet was something tangible I could do.

I stocked up on fruit and asked Joel not to snack in front of Sydney on foods she wasn't allowed to eat. She didn't seem bothered that the bag of Goldfish was suddenly off limits as long as there was a plate of baby carrots, cucumber and apple slices and rolls of turkey in front of her.

The hardest day was the first one. When Sydney was in preschool, it seemed like there were birthday parties for her classmates every time we turned around. And wouldn't you know it, another child was turning five, and Sydney was invited. Normally that would be a good thing, an enjoyable celebration. But I dreaded the party, which, of course, was complete with a huge wheat-filled birthday cake and a donkey piñata filled with unsafe candy.

I had talked with Sydney beforehand and explained in simple terms that gluten was very likely the cause of her stomachaches. As a sweet and compliant child, she was eager to do the right thing. It was just hard having to watch all the other kids eat huge slices of a three-layer birthday cake right under her nose.

Sydney took some of her frustration out on the piñata and managed to be the first child to whack a hole in the side of the donkey. Candy went flying across the floor, and the circle of kids screamed and dove on it. Sydney pulled her blindfold off just in time to grab a few pieces. She looked at the brightly wrapped candy, then, knowing it might not be safe, quietly handed the pieces to me. There were a few tears on the ride home, and I promised Sydney I would find a treat for her to enjoy—one that wouldn't cause a stomachache.

It was after Sydney's dinner and bath that night that the most amazing thing happened. I watched her grow tired as I read to her. This was rare. When I said "Goodnight," and turned out the light, Sydney closed her eyes and fell asleep. She slept through the entire night and didn't wake up until the next morning. This was a first! Well, almost. She had slept through the night a few times in her life, but usually only after an extended period of sleepless nights. To say that I had grown used to expecting her cries to wake me in the middle of the night was an understatement. If it didn't happen, I worried. Suddenly, a full night of sleep. At 7:30 a.m. I checked on Sydney because I was used to her bounding out of bed by 6 a.m. Was it a coincidence? Had gluten been the culprit that had been disturbing her, keeping her awake night after night?

I didn't know the answers for sure. But as a seriously sleep-deprived mom, I couldn't help but note this change. The evidence was enough to make me keep feeding her plates of fruit, vegetables and turkey. And I watched her closely.

Dr. S

$\mathcal{A}$fter two weeks had passed, Joel and I drove into town again with our daughter. My stomach was tight as we navigated the tree-lined streets of Charlotte. We were possibly on the brink of finally discovering what was going on with Sydney. Yet, we had another doctor to meet, the gastroenterologist who would perform Sydney's endoscopy.

When we arrived, a nurse escorted us back to Dr. S's office. I handed him a letter I had typed up about Sydney's history. Even though she'd heard about them plenty of times, I didn't like discussing her symptoms over and over in front of her. On the page, I described her years of severe constipation, lack of energy and sleeplessness. I also included the fact that I had put her on a gluten-free diet for the past two weeks, and we had seen amazing changes. Not only was she sleeping through the night, but she had more energy; her stomachaches had vanished, and she was no longer ravenous right after dinner. All hopeful signs.

Dr. S glanced through what I had written, then gave us a medical definition of celiac disease: "Celiac is a digestive disorder. Everyone's small intestine is lined with villi, tiny finger-like projections that absorb nutrients from the food we eat." Dr. S held up his own fingers and wiggled them. "There are thousands of villi per square inch, which greatly increase the surface area of the small intestine for food absorption. When someone with celiac eats gluten, it triggers an immune response, which causes the body to attack the small intestine and damage these villi." Dr. S bent his fingers so only his knuckles were showing. "Over time, the villi get blunted and shortened, so they're no longer able to absorb nutrients. The only way for these villi to heal is to stop ingesting gluten, which means any food with wheat, barley or rye."

Dr. S paused and looked me in the eye before continuing. "You understand this is a lifelong condition."

I nodded. Sydney, who had been sitting on my lap during this discourse, leaned her head back against my chest and yawned. I wondered what, if anything, she was taking in. I motioned to Joel to hand me a magazine for her to look at.

The doctor went on to explain "secondary lactose intolerance," something I only vaguely understood. He said people with celiac disease are typically unable to digest dairy products because the lining of their gut is so damaged that they no longer have enough lactase, an enzyme necessary to digest a type of milk sugar. This causes stomachaches, gas and bloating. However, once someone stops eating gluten and the villi are restored, he or she can often eat dairy.

I took a deep breath, trying to absorb every bit of information.

Dr. S swiveled on his stool, took a glance at Sydney's chart and began leading us through the procedure. "She'll need an endoscopy. It's the gold standard for testing for celiac," he said. He described how our daughter would be "put under," and a thin tube with a camera on one end would be inserted through her throat, into her esophagus and stomach, down her digestive tract and into her small intestine. Once there, the doctor would take several tiny samples from a few different locations in the small intestine to see if there was any scarring. He said there were no nerve endings in the lining of the small intestine, so the procedure would be painless. After the samples were studied, we would know for sure whether Sydney had celiac disease or not.

I looked down at Sydney. She was patting a tabby in a cat food advertisement.

The doctor asked if Sydney was on a gluten-free diet. I nodded. "Yes, for the past two weeks." I wondered if he had actually read the letter I had so painstakingly written.

36

"Put her back on her regular diet," Dr. S said.

What? Feed my daughter the poison that had been making her sick for the past five years? He had to be crazy! "But she's been feeling so … so good," I stammered.

"The test is more reliable when the patient is eating gluten," Dr. S answered matter-of-factly.

"Can I just give her a little bit?" I was already calculating how I could give her the tiniest bit of wheat in a mostly gluten-free diet. There was no way I wanted her to feel sick again.

"She needs to have several servings a day. Give her at least one piece of bread at every meal. We want to know for sure what's going on in there."

I let out my breath and closed my eyes. Inside I was groaning. I was going to have to give my daughter food that I was pretty sure would harm her. The idea of it made me feel physically ill. Two more weeks of gluten. I was now counting down the days.

As expected, those two weeks were horrific. For me. Sydney was thrilled to see food that had previously vanished from the table reappear. She couldn't wait to eat a roll with dinner again. I turned away as she ate cereal, toast, pasta, crackers, cookies, cake—all filled with gluten. I couldn't watch. The first day was the worst. As soon as she finished breakfast, she was back on the couch, holding her stomach. During the first week, her energy waned, she was irritable and constipated. There were dark smudges under her eyes again as she woke throughout the night. Her ravenous appetite returned, reminding me that whatever she was eating was no longer nourishing her.

Sydney quickly adapted to this unhealthy state. After all, it had been the norm for her for most of her life. But I had seen a glimpse of a new healthful energy in my daughter, and I despised, with everything in me, seeing it doused by a poison named gluten.

Endoscopy

*I*n the predawn hours, Joel and I are quiet as we drive through the empty streets to the hospital. Our five-year-old (the size of a three-and-a-half-year-old) sits quietly, her head leaning against the side of her car seat, her eyes open wide as she hugs BearBear to her chest. The doctor said after the procedure she would most likely nap for the rest of the day.

As we near the hospital complex, streetlights shine into the car. Joel and I have always handled these kinds of things differently. In his jovial way, he likes to talk about the procedure, imagine what it might feel like and what could go wrong. The night before I asked him to filter his words because I didn't want him to unintentionally scare Sydney. I had told her in general terms what would happen, but I spent most of my time reassuring her that we would be with her (or right outside the door), and that she would be asleep during the procedure.

"Will it hurt?" Sydney's small voice asks from the back seat.

Joel and I lock eyes for a moment. Before he can give our daughter his realistic take on how it will feel, I speak up.

"Not a bit, honey," I say. "You won't feel a thing. The doctor will give you something to make you sleepy, and when you wake up, it will all be over."

"And we'll be on our way to Wendy's for a Frosty!" Joel adds. I squeeze Joel's hand in silent affirmation. Frosty's contain dairy, but *they are gluten free and one of Sydney's favorite treats. Since she's been eating gluten these past two weeks, she might as well have one more day of dairy. She could look forward to the soft ice cream, and maybe it would be soothing to her digestive tract.*

In the rearview mirror, I see Sydney smiling. "I can't wait for my Frosty!" she says. "I'm hungry."

"I know, Sweetie. As soon as we're done, we'll get you something good to eat."

The night before, as I was getting Sydney ready for bed, I asked her if she wanted to bring BearBear with her. She thought about it for a moment, then told me she would take him in the car with her but leave him in the car seat. "I don't want to lose him in the hospital," she said.

"He'll be waiting for you," I said giving her a hug.

We are only in the waiting room a few minutes before the nurse calls us back. We follow her to a small room with a curtain around it. There is a hospital bed surrounded by various medical devices. Leaning against the pillow is a stuffed animal with a tag around its neck which reads: "A Comfort Bear for You." I lift Sydney onto the bed and tears spring to my eyes as she immediately enfolds the bear in her arms.

The nurse takes Sydney's temperature and blood pressure and says she'll be back with something to drink. "It tastes like Kool-Aid and it will make you sleepy."

I consider explaining that we don't give Sydney things like Kool-Aid, that her diet has been restricted, and that's the reason we're here in the hospital. But I let the moment pass.

The nurse returns with a paper cup of red liquid. Sydney sniffs it and takes a tiny taste. "Mmm..." she says, then drinks it down. The nurse tells her to lie down on the bed. As Sydney's eyes close, the nurse takes my daughter's tiny hand and inserts an IV needle into the back of it and tapes it down.

Sydney's small body takes up only a third of the bed. My heart aches for her. This shouldn't be happening. She shouldn't be in a hospital— enduring needles, being anesthetized, preparing for a procedure where a tube will be forced down her throat and threaded through her digestive tract. I want to pick her up, hold her tightly against my chest and run as fast as I can away from this place.

But I step back as the nurse lifts the side rails of the hospital bed in preparation for transport. She glances at me as I reach toward Sydney and stroke her arm. Her cheeks are slightly flushed, and her skin feels like rose petals. She is so young and tender, so fresh and vulnerable. If I could trade places with her I would.

The nurse releases the wheels on the gurney with her foot and nudges the bed forward with her hip as she pushes the curtain back. She points the way to the waiting room. "I'll take good care of her."

I can tell from his face that Joel feels as forlorn as I do, watching our daughter being wheeled down the hall. I squeeze my husband's hand and feel the heat in his skin.

After what felt like an endless time in the waiting room, the doctor appeared before us. I searched his face for news, but it was inscrutable. Had we put Sydney through this procedure needlessly? Was he about to shake his head and say he was sorry, there wasn't enough evidence to diagnose her? I had heard nothing definitive for so long from any doctor that I couldn't imagine anything beyond another dead-end road, another disappointment. A morning show blared on the television; people around us flipped magazine pages; behind a glass wall, the receptionist's head was bent, and her eyes were downcast as if even she couldn't bear to see our reaction to the doctor's lack of news.

Dr. S cleared his throat. "Your daughter's doing fine. We took a sample of tissue from several places in her small intestine…."

Yeah, yeah, yeah. I know that. Come on, tell us something we don't know. The words inside my head clambered to get out, but I held myself back.

"We have to send the samples out for testing."

I sighed. This just meant more waiting. More time in this impossible state of limbo. "Can you tell us anything?" I pleaded.

The doctor looked me in the eye. His cheery, lighthearted manner seemed in contrast to whatever news he was carrying. What must it be like for him to deliver news to parents on a daily basis? Or to face the questions of parents when he had nothing to share?

A serious expression flashed across the doctor's face. "Your daughter has severe scarring in her small intestine. I don't need to wait for the tests to tell you this. I can say, without a doubt, that she has celiac disease."

His words made my mind go blank. "Scarring?" I paused and took a breath. "Severe?"

Was this what I had wanted...a diagnosis? But not if it meant my sweet girl was *scarred*. I thought there might be a little redness, some irritation, not "severe scarring."

The doctor went on to explain that this type of scarring, which was consistent with celiac disease, meant the villi lining her intestinal tract had been worn smooth from years of eating gluten. This was keeping her from being able to absorb nutrients. Despite eating multiple times a day, our daughter was literally starving because her food wasn't nourishing her.

This is why she was small; *this* is why she was hungry all the time; *this* is why she had trouble sleeping. Part of me already knew this. But to hear confirmation from the doctor was different. All the cards were falling into place. I felt dizzy trying to contain my emotions. A sense of relief and affirmation for all the days, weeks, months and years of struggling to understand what was wrong with my daughter's health. Knowing deep down there was something despite the myriad times my concerns had been dismissed, rejected, even ridiculed.

But at the same time, a yawning chasm opened within me as I took in the information that Sydney's small intestine had been damaged. Scarred, inflamed, injured. If I knew in my own gut that something was off, why hadn't I been able to catch it, fix it, save her from all these years of pain? She had suffered, and I hadn't been able to stop it. Could I ever forgive myself?

But now we had proof. We knew what was wrong. We could begin to fix it. My body itched to start the healing process, to go out and find every crumb of wheat that might be in our home and banish it forever.

Relief. Guilt. Sorrow. Acceptance. Determination. These were just a few of the emotions swirling within me.

"You can go back and see her in a few minutes," Dr. S said, "as soon as the anesthesia wears off. She'll be sleepy the rest of the day. But you'll want to keep an eye on her to make sure she has no adverse reactions."

Joel and I stood up to shake the doctor's hand as he turned to leave. My legs trembled, and I saw tiny spots where his face had been. I took a deep breath and my vision cleared. It was time to see our girl.

Sydney wiped her eyes groggily as Joel and I entered the room. The head of her hospital bed was raised, and her new stuffed bear was nestled in her arms. Her face brightened when she saw us, and I rushed over to give her a hug. Her body was warm and soft as a fresh-baked muffin.

"You did so well, Sweetie!" I exclaimed.

Sydney gave me a sleepy smile. She looked at the back of her hand where the IV had been taped. "Is it over?" she asked.

"It's over!" both Joel and I responded.

"Time for your Frosty!" said Joel.

"Did the little camera go inside me?" She rubbed her arm.

"It did," I said. "And it was very helpful. The doctor figured out why your tummy has been sore. And we know how to fix it."

Sydney's beautiful eyes opened wider. She hugged her bear to her chest. "Is BearBear in the car?"

"Yes, Sweetie," I said, gathering her in my arms. "He's waiting for you."

After the Endoscopy

*I*t was only later that we learned Sydney thought the IV was "the little camera." She had imagined it going up through her arm, down her throat and into her small intestine, taking photos all along the way. She wondered how a camera could actually do that, and she noticed happily, after she woke up, that her arm wasn't sore. I laughed later thinking about this because I was sure I had done such a good job of explaining in "kid terms" what was going to happen to her. Either I left out some things or her imagination took over.

On the way home, Sydney had a large Frosty, which seemed like a lot to me, until I remembered that she still wasn't absorbing nutrients and wouldn't be able to until the villi in her gut began to heal.

When we got home, I fed Sydney a late lunch and kept expecting her to drift off to sleep, so I could grab a quick nap. My eyes were bloodshot from nights of not sleeping well, and today's alarm had gone off before 5 a.m. Every part of me felt ragged from the emotional pinball that had been going on inside me for the last several hours.

Napping wasn't typical for Sydney. But she'd been up as long as I had, and her little body had been pumped full of anesthesia. If Joel or I had been sedated for an endoscopy, we'd barely be able to function, much less keep our eyes open for the rest of the day.

But not Sydney. She was full of energy. More than usual. Can you say firecracker? She was climbing on the furniture and taking flying leaps off of it, something she normally didn't do. She begged me to set up an obstacle course out of pillows and blocks in the living room, and she wanted me to do it with her. I told her I would do it once, then Mom had to rest.

When I stretched out on the couch and told her to pick a favorite book, she snuggled against me for a moment. Then, as if some internal spinner was going off inside her, she started moving again. Maybe she was sugared up from the Frosty; maybe she sensed the intense emotion of the day, or maybe she was just having an unusual reaction to the anesthesia.

Eventually, she gathered all her stuffed animals (and she had a LOT of them) and laid them side by side on the floor. She covered up their bodies with her old baby blankets and dug out her doctor's kit. After examining the animals and listening to their hearts with her stethoscope, she diagnosed most of them with tummy aches. She gave them shots and told them they would have to drink something red. "We'll put a little camera in you to find out what's going on," she told them.

I had work to do—reading and researching about celiac, clearing out cupboards, shopping for gluten-free food, creating menus for family meals, etc.—but I couldn't pull myself away, despite how tired we both were. I kept waiting for the doctor's words to come true, for Sydney to get sleepy, for her to drop from exhaustion, so that I could throw myself into this work. But it never happened. Sydney would be gluten free from now on, but she still wasn't ready to nap.

Perhaps I should have followed our normal routine. I could have taken Sydney into her room, read a few books to her and told her it was rest time, that Mommy was going upstairs to read and rest also, and that she could come up and find me when the digital clock read a certain time.

But nothing about this day felt normal. It was already way past naptime. And I didn't want to leave her. It wasn't just that I wanted to observe her (as the doctor had suggested) for any reactions to her procedure. I wanted to feast my eyes—even if they were red and burning—on her sweet little form. Her precious face, her energy, her Sydney-ness were so beautiful. Despite this condition she had lived with all her life, it hadn't dimmed her incredible spirit one iota. She was strong and full of courage; she emanated light; her lifeforce seemed to sparkle. I couldn't get enough of her.

The Learning Curve

*B*efore Sydney's endoscopy, the doctor had told us that if he discovered celiac as the cause of our daughter's symptoms, we'd have to eliminate every trace of gluten from Sydney's diet. He said even a speck of wheat, barley or rye could cause damage to her intestinal tract. Dr. S also cautioned us to keep Sydney off dairy for several months, until the villi in her gut had time to heal.

It's hard to understand the enormity of a change like this if you haven't been through it. As the mother and the main gatekeeper for all the food in our home, I took the challenge seriously. For years, I had watched Sydney suffer, knowing that something was wrong, but not understanding the root cause. Finally, *this* was something I could do. I would be the Mother Tiger, wiping out every trace of gluten in her life.

I took over all the grocery shopping. (Joel had begun doing some of it after I was ordered on bedrest eight weeks before Sydney was born, and I had gladly let him continue.) But no more. For one thing, Joel was used to shopping from a list I produced for him several times a week. He didn't have the patience to study every label looking for words that might denote gluten. Shopping trips grew from ten-minute errands to two-hour, headache-inducing excursions as I scanned each and every canned or boxed food.

I had poured over website after website, jotting down the places where gluten could hide. Words like maltodextrin and modified food starch could signify wheat. *What? It doesn't even say gluten? How could that be?* But I learned that wheat was often the "modified food" or one of the starches used in these ingredients. Gluten might also be found in artificial flavors and colors, citric acid, emulsifiers, glycerides, stabilizers and so many more things. What made it extra tricky was that gluten wasn't *always* found in these ingredients, but it *might* be. In addition, there were bags of gluten-free snacks—chips, cookies, nuts—that were produced in facilities that also packaged wheat and other allergens. Did that make them unsafe? Possibly. No one could tell me for sure. It depended on the product; it depended on the person.

I learned there were degrees of sensitivity. Some people with celiac could handle foods with a touch of natural flavorings, while the same ingredient would set off an awful reaction (hours of throwing up or digestive upset) in others. Some people were so sensitive that even a kiss on the cheek from someone who had recently eaten gluten could cause intense swelling.

The last thing I wanted to do was experiment with my daughter in the hopes that we happened upon the right safety measures. Her intestines had already been scarred. I didn't want to further the damage. The only option was to eliminate gluten in every way I could.

Dr. S had told us to bring Sydney back to his office in six months for another checkup, admonishing us that no matter how hard we tried, our daughter would get some gluten in her system. He said she would need bloods tests twice a year. They would tell us how much and what kind of exposure to wheat she'd had.

I thought to myself, "No way. I'm not going to put my daughter through needless blood tests. She had been a champion, already enduring so much more than the typical child. Blood tests apparently keep some people from cheating (and may be a wise protocol for most people to follow). But Sydney was five. She ate what we gave her, and she trusted us. She didn't want to feel bad. And it wasn't like we were going to just *try* to remove gluten from her diet. I was already one hundred percent committed. This wasn't a choice. I wouldn't need blood tests to confirm we were following the program or to know we'd made a mistake. We'd see evidence of our success or failure in Sydney. Her growth, her sleep, her energy levels.

Besides, if anyone could eliminate gluten from Sydney's diet, I knew I could. As an editor by trade, I had an eagle eye and was used to looking out for anything that didn't belong or might be out of place.

Part of me felt as if I'd been born to do this job, to scour our days for any stray crumbs of gluten, pouncing on and eradicating them when they were discovered.

At the same time, another part of me mourned. The flood of what Sydney could no longer enjoy overtook me. No more cookies, cakes, pizza, crackers, toast…everything that …*well*… tasted good. Was food even worth eating if you couldn't enjoy your favorite treats?

And what *could* she eat? The advice that was repeated on several celiac websites was "Shop on the perimeter of the grocery store." That meant fruit, vegetables, eggs, meat." Okay, strawberries, bananas, apples, broccoli, green beans, carrots, hamburgers, chicken…. There's nothing wrong with those things. But to eat *only* those things… *forever*! What about dessert? After all, it was my primary food group when I was a kid.

It didn't take long for me to discover that desserts were the easiest things to find in the ironically named "health food stores." Gluten-free cookies, candy, box mixes of brownies and cake were readily available. But not the foods I longed to share with my daughter like my mother's wonderful Johnny Marzetti (a dish piled full of noodles, tomato sauce and cheese), the calzones we purchased at our favorite Italian hole-in-the-wall restaurant, the Friday night pizzas we ordered when no one felt like cooking or the four-inch high sandwiches Joel and I were used to indulging in on the weekends.

Eating out was one of the first things to go. Surprisingly, I hardly gave it a thought. What I wouldn't do for myself, I would gladly do for Sydney. I would happily give up restaurants, even though they had nourished me for the better part of my life, if what they served might harm my daughter. And, just as important, I didn't want her to suffer by having to watch her parents indulge in something she couldn't eat.

But still, questions remained: How would I feed her? What would we eat?

I say "we" because almost instantaneously I made the decision that if Sydney was going gluten free, I would do the same. It was only fair, and a small sacrifice for a mother to make if it would help to ease Sydney's transition. If she had to face life without wheat, I would be beside her.

Joel and I discussed the issue of gluten in our home. For Sydney's sake, I wanted to get rid of as much of it as possible, and segregate any gluten-filled foods, so she wouldn't accidentally eat them. My plan was to eventually eradicate every speck of wheat from our home. But while I wanted to keep wheat and its poisonous cousins away from Sydney, I knew it would be a process and take some time to clear it out completely.

Joel was more than willing to eat gluten-free snacks and meals at home. He would eat anything I put in front of him, actually. But he wasn't ready to commit to a completely gluten-free lifestyle. That was fine with me. We didn't know if either of us were sensitive to gluten, though I had learned that celiac ran in families, so it wouldn't have surprised me. Besides, it was a lot easier for me to throw a frozen pot pie made with a wheat crust on a separate pan in the oven for Joel, than to make two gluten-free pot pies from scratch. (Two instead of one, because my husband ate a lot more than Sydney and me, and it was critical to have leftovers.)

As a mother to my long-awaited daughter, I figured the best way I could support Sydney would be to make going gluten free as normal as possible. If we ate the same meals, she wouldn't feel like she was alone. One day, she would have to face a world that was full of gluten on her own. But for now, within our family, we could provide a safe haven, where she wouldn't have to dodge gluten at every turn. Our refrigerator, our cupboards, our breakfasts, lunches and dinners would be gluten free.

Here at home, instead of being different, Sydney would be a leader and the reason that Joel and I were making healthier food choices. We could set the tone and be thankful for the changes in our lives instead of focusing on what we were missing.

My husband has often said that I'm an idealist, and it's not always a compliment. Yes, I can get on my high horse and ride to the tune of my own ideals, imagining a beautiful outcome for everything and everybody. The way it works out in my mind is lovely and inspiring.

But it's probably no surprise that Joel took a bit longer than I did to embrace this change in our way of eating. And, of course, life is always more complicated than my idealistic daydreams.

Not all parents are willing to give up gluten for their child. Nor should they necessarily. Especially if they have other children who don't have celiac. It's a judgment call, and every family is unique and will hopefully make decisions with the best interest of all in mind. Children who have celiac, even those who live in an allergen-free home, will grow up one day and have to experience the real world where others are sitting beside them devouring gluten-filled pizza or kindly offering them a homemade cookie made with sugar, butter, molasses and wheat flour. There is no way to completely insulate your child. If there was, I would have found it. So, with the understanding that parents know their children best, it is important to remember there are many ways forward.

Visiting the RDN

*O*ne of the first things we did after Sydney's endoscopy was to make an appointment with a registered dietitian nutritionist (RDN). Dr. S gave us the name of a woman—Pat Fogarty—who he'd worked with for several years. Her daughter had celiac disease, and Pat was well known in Charlotte area gluten-free circles. Who knew those things even existed? But as I researched celiac, Pat's name came up time and again.

Joel would have been happy to have me go solo on this appointment, but I felt it was important for him to join me as part of our on-going education about celiac. From my reading, I was learning that his laissez faire attitude about occasional wheat exposures could get us into trouble. Rather than continue to harp on him (as I'd been doing already, with no effect), I figured this issue was serious enough that he needed to hear it from someone else.

I arranged for a babysitter to watch Sydney while we made the fifty-minute drive to south Charlotte to the nutritionist's house. As this was the first time Joel and I had been alone together for weeks, we joked about it being a date.

On the drive down, we talked about what we'd just been through—the intensity of the endoscopy, the relief of finally getting a diagnosis, the hope of watching our daughter heal, the overwhelming task of shifting to a completely gluten-free diet and the acknowledgment of the enormity of this change. Correction. I talked, and Joel listened. And I talked some more, and he listened. And so on.

Suddenly, we were almost there. Joel pulled into the nutritionist's neighborhood and slowed down to look for her house number. It was an upscale subdivision with large oak trees and big brick houses. I found myself thinking of the nutritionist's daughter, imagining her playing outside, riding her bike. In my mind, she was normal, lucky, in fact, that she had a mom who could protect her from the scourge of gluten. Maybe I could offer that same gift to Sydney.

Pat met us at the door and invited us into her kitchen. The table and countertops were lined with flattened cardboard boxes of various shapes and sizes, which I soon realized were all empty packages of gluten-free food. Pat was kind and professional. She invited us to sit down and offered us something to drink. She gave us several handouts as she asked about our daughter.

Pat gave us an overview of how to be gluten free in a gluten-filled world, including shopping on the perimeter of the grocery store. But she didn't stop there. She gave us the names of the best health food stores, provided recipes for certain dishes and substitutions for ingredients that were off limits; she offered great tips, such as "Passover is a great time to find gluten-free goodies at a good price in the regular supermarkets." She listed the names of a few restaurants that offered gluten-free fare, with the caveat that some places were okay for those who were gluten intolerant but not safe for people with celiac.

She took us on a tour through the boxes in her kitchen. There were various brands of gluten-free flour, crackers, pasta, and cookie and cake mixes. Many of the labels were unfamiliar, and Pat gave me the names and addresses of companies and websites where certain foods could be ordered. At the time, most of these items were not available at regular grocery stores.

I was amazed at all the options, but cautious too, knowing that neither Sydney nor I were very adventurous when it came to trying new foods.

Pat told us about her daughter. She was eleven, six years older than Sydney, and highly reactive to gluten. The tiniest amount would set off her symptoms—a cycle of digestive issues including vomiting and diarrhea. Her daughter had a circle of friends; she went to the movies, had sleepovers (these things were encouraging). She knew what brands of popcorn were safe, and Pat provided gluten-free lunches and bags of snacks for her when she went out. Yet, in the midst of "normal living," I heard that her daughter still got sick. Just a few days ago, she'd had an exposure. It didn't happen often, just once or twice a year, when she encountered cross contamination with gluten at a restaurant or in social situations. But it was more than I wanted to hear. Even though her daughter had been diagnosed with celiac several years ago, *and* she had a mother who was a nutritionist, she wasn't completely insulated from the dangers of gluten.

The enormity of what we were facing with Sydney washed over me again. While I could help protect Sydney, if she was going to live a normal life, I couldn't remove all the risks. No one could.

I was glad Joel was here. I was the one who would prepare most, if not all, of our meals, especially in the beginning. But it would take both of us doing our best to keep Sydney healthy and safe from gluten exposures.

If I thought about it (which I tried not to), as Sydney's mom, I was responsible for building a new way of eating for our family from the ground up. At least eighty percent of the food my daughter had existed on (and probably ninety-five percent of the food she truly loved) was suddenly off limits, including most of what she used to eat during Thanksgiving, Christmas and Easter holidays.

Joel and I spent almost two hours with Pat, and I was reluctant to leave. I had asked questions, listened intently, wrote notes. In her sunny, welcoming kitchen, it seemed possible that I could provide meals for Sydney and nourish her properly. But at home? If I was bold and dedicated, I could start by looking up recipes, trying to recreate some of what I'd grown up enjoying. I was bold (to a degree) and dedicated (to the extreme). But with my history as a noncook, I knew it wouldn't be easy.

Pat encouraged and fortified me with plenty of information to get me started. She even gave me a bag of gluten-free chocolate chip mix. She put me on her mailing list and gave me her email so that I could contact her as new questions arose.

However, by the time Joel and I got back in the car, my head was pounding. I'd been listening so intently, trying to glean every bit of information that I could get from Pat that I'd ignored the waves of emotion that were welling up inside me. Despite feeling hopeful, I found myself in tears on the way home, blubbering to Joel that it was all too much, "This is too hard! I have no idea what I'm doing. How can I cook for Sydney if I don't know how to cook for myself? What if I can't find enough food to feed her? What if she gets an exposure and we don't know it, and her intestinal tract stays inflamed? What if she gets sick?" I just wanted our little girl to be safe.

Joel was wise enough to let me cry it out. He gently reassured me that we would do this together. That, yes, while he knew that clearing our lives of the dreaded gluten was going to be my responsibility, he would fully back me. Despite the fact that he wasn't quite ready to give up gluten himself yet, I knew I could count on him.

Jean

$\mathcal{M}$ y commitment to providing a gluten-free lifestyle for our family never wavered. Yet, particularly during the first weeks and months, I felt overwhelmed. My idealism went out the window, along with any confidence in my ability to provide tasty meals. Even with the excellent advice and resources of the RDN, I still had to reconstruct my thinking. I was used to living as a noncook, and I couldn't keep the questions from circling in my head: How would we eat? How could I possibly find food to feed my family? Would starvation set in?

It's a challenge to totally re-enter that mental space because now (after more than ten years of eating this way) I've set myself up with enough cupboard ingredients, basic recipes and meals to feel secure. I know how to prowl the aisles of the grocery store, pick up staples of meat, eggs, veggies and fruit on the perimeter, selectively stalk the inner aisles for nuts, almond and coconut milk, and the few boxed goods that are safe.

Back then, gluten-free food was so much less available. Even the term "gluten free" was hardly recognized. People would look at us funny when we mentioned it. There were no gluten-free boxes of cookies or cake in regular grocery stores; gluten-free pasta or treats were relegated to the health food stores. It was a rare restaurant that served gluten-free food or offered allergy-free menus.

Joel continued to straddle the line, indulging in his usual gluten-filled diet when he was out of the house, but happily devouring gluten-free food around our dinner table when there was enough to share.

My dilemma was always the next meal—tonight's food...and tomorrow's lunch...and dinner and the one after that and after that. How would I feed us all?

I purchased a gluten-free shopping guide. It broke down foods by category and listed brands that were gluten free. Unfortunately, I'd never heard of most of the brands or our local stores didn't carry them. Every shopping trip left me holding my head in despair. For a noncook like me, this wasn't getting any easier.

Jean, a dear friend, heard me moaning about the challenges of feeding my family and invited me into her kitchen. I remember sitting on a barstool at her island. She let me go on about my gluten-free troubles for a little bit before whipping out a pad of paper and a pen.

"What do you like to eat?" she asked, studying me over her reading glasses.

Woefully, I shared how I'd always been a picky eater, and my daughter was no less so. Joel, fortunately, would eat almost anything I put in front of him.

"Well, let's start with a list of foods that you and Sydney *will* eat," she said. "Chicken?" she asked raising her eyebrows.

I wanted to keep complaining, but with Jean's earnest, kind-hearted face before me, I had to muster some maturity. "Yes, chicken, hamburger and steak for main meals," I acquiesced. "Broccoli, string beans and salads for sides." These were all safe. But after a lifetime of eating out or dining on frozen, boxed meals, they felt incomplete.

"How about bread?" Jean asked.

I shook my head and grimaced. "Have you tasted that stuff?" I hadn't found any gluten-free bread that was even close to palatable. But I would keep looking.

"Spaghetti?"

"I could give rice pasta a try," I said slowly. "Maybe the change in taste and texture won't be noticeable under spaghetti sauce." I gave a little smirk. Oh, and the spaghetti sauce needed to be gluten free. I should be able to find that, I thought to myself. I had jotted down the names of gluten-free pasta sauce when I was with Pat. Maybe I could do this.

"Potatoes?" Jean continued.

Yes. I nodded. I could cook them and even stuff them, though I didn't admit to the stuffing part. I was not about to fully embrace the art of cooking.

"Tacos?"

"I guess so," I admitted. There were tortillas made from corn I could use, and the nutritionist had told me about a gluten-free taco mix, if I wanted to get fancy.

"Eggs?"

"Well, Joel and Sydney like them scrambled," I responded half-heartedly. Part of my gloom was simply that I hadn't fully accepted the fact that my life had changed, and I wasn't happy about it. In my zeal to provide healthy, gluten-free food for my daughter, I hadn't given myself time to process my own grief. I wasn't just giving up all things wheat-related, but my persona—the woman who spent her time and energy focused on writing and poetry, the woman who apparently had taken pride in rarely making a home-cooked meal—was being turned inside out. I just needed to pout. "I suppose I could make an egg casserole," I said slowly, and added begrudgingly, "with gluten-free ingredients."

Casseroles were one of the dishes I'd been silently missing. Gone were the casseroles of my childhood. My mother's Johnny Marzetti, creamy chicken and noodle casserole, etc., etc. Even my old standby—Campbell's soup—had gluten in it! No longer could I glibly dump a few ingredients into a dish and have an easy meal and leftovers. It just wasn't fair, I whined to myself.

Jean studied me with soft brown eyes. "It's hard, isn't it?" Her kindness brought a lump to my throat. I nodded, and she enfolded me in a hug.

Stepping back, she continued, "So, what about snacks?"

While I wanted to prolong my moping, I forgave Jean her persistence. She was a deeply compassionate friend. She wanted to help me because she knew I was worried about feeding my family, and she wanted me to be well-fortified on every front. She was willing to wade through my resistance and self-defeating attitude to help me find a path forward.

"Popcorn?"

"Yes. But not all popcorn...." With a frown on my face I explained that there were only a couple of microwaveable brands that were safe.

"Fruit?"

"Yes, but how much fruit can one person eat?" I rolled my eyes and fake-moaned before finally starting to laugh at myself. I knew I wasn't making this easy for her.

"Crackers?" she went on.

More moaning from me. It would be a long and intense search before I could find crackers that were edible, much less tasty, I told her.

"And what about desserts?"

Yes, I could make them from scratch. But having avoided the kitchen for most of my adult life, how many hours could I bear to be within range of a hot oven?

Jean talked me off one cliff and then the next. There were fruit cups that were safe that I could pack in Sydney's lunch. I could bake one large batch of brownies or cookies and freeze them, so I could pull out treats on a regular basis (without having to constantly bake). I told her about the gluten-free cookie mix the nutritionist had given me.

With Jean's help, I left her house with a list of meals, snacks and desserts that I could produce for a week. It was a lifeline. Something I would use to help me and my family survive the first few months of living gluten free.

My GF Journey

A few months after Sydney's endoscopy, I requested that I be tested for celiac during my annual physical. For most of my life, I had experienced symptoms that I now realized could be attributed to gluten intolerance: bloating, diarrhea, fatigue, brain fog, achiness in my joints, periods of mild depression, etc.

Like my daughter, my blood test came back inconclusive. But I'd already made up my mind. I wanted to support Sydney, and after all the reading I'd done about the disease, I was pretty sure I'd feel better changing my diet and getting wheat out of my system. Even back in 2006, some researchers and doctors suspected that eating gluten would negatively impact most people. In 2015, a Harvard study actually proved that exposure to gluten increased intestinal permeability in both celiac and non-celiac patients.[3] Since celiac is a genetic condition that runs in families, I figured at the very least, I probably had gluten intolerance, if not full-blown celiac.

Lest you get the wrong idea about me, I was *not* a gluten-free martyr. It was easier for me to give up traditional bread, pies, cookies and cakes as long as I could replace them with gluten-free versions. I was much more attached to sugar than I was to wheat, barley or rye.

For the most part, I focused on what I *could* eat, not what I couldn't. Unlike Joel, I didn't fixate on pizza or the homemade cakes and pies that lined the tables at our church potluck meals. I did miss having a piece of toast with which to scoop up my scrambled eggs. And I searched long and hard for a pizza crust that would be safe *and* tasty. (Eventually I gave that up because, let's face it, nothing compares to a hot-delivered pizza with a thick, chewy, wheat-filled crust.)

Certain foods like brownies and cookies could be replicated without gluten. Food connoisseurs said the texture was different, that rice flour didn't compare to the fluffy stickiness of wheat flour, but most of the time I didn't care, as long as the sweetness was still there.

In fact, in some ways it felt freeing to leave all those breaded things behind. I'd never craved them, and now I had a good excuse not to eat them if they were served to me. I could pick and choose the food I really wanted to eat—the ultimate joy for the picky eater.

Going gluten free didn't have an immediate impact on my health. From what I'd read, it would take at least four to six weeks for my body to respond and begin healing. In fact, the improvement was so subtle, I couldn't be sure anything was happening. Experiencing the gradual absence of symptoms was a tricky thing to quantify.

In some ways, it felt as if my body was running cleaner, my digestive processes were smooth. My mind was clearer. I didn't seem to have as many little aches and pains. My mood was better. Or was I just imagining these things?

Early on, the biggest change happened when I slipped up and accidentally ate wheat. The first time it happened, I had popped a piece of honey candy into my mouth. It was labelled "all-natural," and I was used to splurging on a few pieces after a headache-inducing trip to the health food store. I just assumed the candy was gluten free. That day, I bought a small bag of these candies (at a ridiculously high price—but, oh well, it was worth it, I thought) and treated myself after lunch and dinner for a few days.

Suddenly, I was waking in the middle of the night. My gut was uncomfortable, as if I'd eaten something that didn't agree with me (which I had). It hit me that for a couple of days, I'd felt a creeping sense of irritation—both physical and mental. I'd brushed it off during the daylight hours, but after midnight there wasn't much else to do but ponder the possibilities. I checked off what I'd eaten for breakfast, lunch and dinner. Scrambled eggs, salad, rice, a hamburger and green beans for dinner and a couple of handfuls of gluten-free tortilla chips. Nothing unusual.

Then I remembered the little bag of honey candy. No way! I'd just had two small pieces that day, and three the day before. I got out of bed to look up the ingredients on my computer. Since I couldn't sleep, I might as well do some research. There in the ingredients was malt syrup. Malt was a word I recognized as a hidden source of gluten. It was usually made from barley, one of the grains known for containing gluten.

I sighed. I didn't feel horribly sick, just off. I could function, but there was a mild drag on all my body processes. But not being able to sleep. That was noticeable. Very noticeable. It was clear my body did not like gluten.

Apparently, these symptoms were something I had lived with my whole life. I had just grown used to feeling this way. Once I identified these reactions to gluten, I was more than happy to leave them behind.

Surprises

I watched Sydney closely as her diet changed. From my reading, I'd learned that children usually heal from intestinal scarring much quicker than adults. It might only take a few weeks for her system to purge five years of gluten. Or, there was a slight chance that she wouldn't heal. Our doctor had warned, and I had read, that a small percentage of people, for unknown reasons, never recover despite being on a gluten-free diet.

I chose to think positively. There was no reason that Sydney shouldn't regain her health. Joel and I were strong and active. Both my family and his had a history of relatively good genes. But Sydney wasn't progressing as I had hoped. Her growth continued at a snail's pace, and even though she was sleeping better (most nights), she still had dark circles under her eyes. Something wasn't right. But I had no idea what it was.

I turned myself inside out trying to find any hidden sources of gluten. Was she being exposed to too much wheat in her preschool classroom? Could gluten be in her cold medicine? In the hand soap or shampoo? I talked with her preschool teachers, spent time online researching every celiac site; I spoke to the pharmacist, called medical companies, sent emails to the nutritionist.

One day, as I followed a rabbit trail of information about hidden sources of gluten, I stumbled upon the fact that most brands of chicken were processed with ingredients that contain wheat. *Chicken*? No way! Chicken was our go-to food. It was on the outer rim of the supermarket. I quickly looked up the brands we typically purchased. Yup, somewhere in the fine print there was "modified food starch" or "processed with wheat." My mind reeled as I thought of the number of times we ate chicken each week.

I hoped that the tiny amount of gluten contained in the processing wasn't enough to cause further harm to Sydney. But I feared it had. From that day on, I only purchased chicken that was "natural and unprocessed" or brands of chicken that were labelled gluten free.

After making this adjustment, it didn't take long before Joel and I began to see real changes in Sydney. It was impossible to know if it was the chicken that made the difference or if her body had simply caught up with this new way of eating. But suddenly, it seemed as if Sydney was growing overnight. And she was! The pants she had worn for the past three years were too short! Were my eyes deceiving me? No. I tracked her growth on a homemade chart on the door of her bedroom. She actually grew an inch in less than a week!

During that summer, Sydney's bloated belly gradually disappeared. As she grew taller, her stomach became flat. She still had a big appetite, which I figured was her body's way of making up for years of malnourishment. But no matter how much she ate, she stayed slim. Over time, she stopped asking for seconds and thirds, and, once in a while, she actually left food on her plate.

Sydney also had new bursts of energy. She no longer just wanted to lie on the couch and read or sit at the table and put together puzzles. She still loved to build train tracks with Joel, but they became more and more elaborate. We spent time at the park where she would swing as high as I could push her, climb the jungle gym, ride her bicycle. The boundaries of her world expanded. And she slept at night.

I could hardly believe my luck. After five years of sleep deprivation, it was hard for me to trust that this would continue. In the beginning, I often woke in the middle of the night expecting to hear a cry. But the house was silent. Sometimes I even tiptoed down to Sydney's bedroom just to witness this miracle. Peeking through the cracked door, I saw my daughter's head nestled into her pillow, heard her exhale soft puffs of air. Sweaty curls no longer clung to her cheeks, and her body wasn't splayed out on top of her comforter. Sydney slept on her side with one arm around BearBear, a blanket pulled up to her chest. She could have been any normal five-year-old.

Despite all the noticeable improvements, I couldn't deny that the transition to a gluten-free lifestyle was hard. More than hard. But it was worth it, especially because of the impact on Sydney's health. But just as I was congratulating myself on our success, I was reminded of the pitfalls that existed everywhere.

One Saturday afternoon, Joel offered to make a run to the health food store with Sydney. I made a detailed shopping list and knew that Joel was looking forward to picking out a special treat for Sydney.

When they got home, I took one look at my daughter's face and knew something was wrong. Her cheeks were pale, and her eyes had a glassy, faraway look. She was not her usual cheerful self.

"Did you find something good at the store?" I asked her.

Sydney nodded, then pressed her body into me.

Joel was unpacking the bags, exuberant about some of their gluten-free finds. "They had a table full of wheat-free stuff!" Joel said. "They had all these gluten-free vendors, and the samples were free!"

"Great!" I said. "Did you check the ingredients?"

"These cookies are fine," Joel said, pulling two boxes of chocolate chip cookies out of the bag. "It says gluten free right on the box."

"No, I meant the stuff on the table."

Joel sighed, exasperated at my meticulous concern. "There was a sign. It said gluten free. I bought a couple of packages of those strawberry strudels. They were delicious, weren't they, Sydney?"

"They were yummy," she said.

One package would have been plenty, I thought to myself. But I knew he liked to spoil Sydney, not to mention he enjoyed treating himself.

"I don't feel good, Mommy." Sydney leaned against me, and I sensed the wave of nausea coming.

I led her into the bathroom, and within a moment whatever she had eaten from "the table" came back up.

Of course, I couldn't be sure if this was from a gluten exposure or if Sydney was coming down with a stomach bug. Unlike the nutritionist's daughter, Sydney had never reacted to gluten with nausea. I learned from the doctor that the cleaner Sydney's diet was, the stronger her system would react to even a tiny speck of wheat.

Sydney threw up twice. She seemed to feel better pretty quickly. I wiped her face with a wet washcloth, and we returned to the kitchen.

"Let me take a look at the package of strudel you bought," I said.

Joel pulled it out of the pantry and handed it to me.

I scanned the ingredients. "Wheat flour! Joel, this says wheat... right here!" I pointed to the label.

Joel's face fell. "Oh, no," he said softly.

"Is this what you ate at the store?" I asked.

Joel nodded, and Sydney looked stricken.

"It wasn't gluten free?" she said. "Da-ad! I thought you said it was."

"The sign said...." Joel knew it didn't matter what the sign said. I could tell he felt awful, so I defended him. "Honey, he thought it was safe. Daddy never would have given you gluten if he'd known. It just shows how careful you have to be."

"I'm never eating anything Dad gives me again," Sydney said.

It didn't take Sydney long to forgive Joel. She adored her father and knew he would never intentionally hurt her. But that day she learned to check the ingredients on anything that anyone offered her, even if it was someone she knew and loved, and they assured her the food was gluten free.

Travel

$\mathcal{N}$ ow what about travel? I didn't let my mind go there. I just couldn't even imagine how we would ever leave home. I mean I needed to be within range of our own pantry and kitchen for three meals a day, not to mention snacks. Anywhere beyond a thirty-minute drive seemed out of the question.

But we had a trip looming that summer. A week at my mother's family summer home in Lake George, New York, over eight hundred miles away. At least there was a house with a kitchen where we would stay. But figuring out thirty-five-plus meals and snacks that would keep us alive, not to mention how and where to purchase that food seemed beyond impossible. And let's not forget eating on the road. No more fast food for us. How would we live?

That first trip practically sent me around the bend. I remember complaining to my husband that "This was supposed to be a vacation!" when, in actuality, I was spending just as many hours as we'd be away, planning for the trip. It was hard enough to come up with a week of meals at home. Suddenly, I had to reproduce those meals (with the same or similar safe ingredients) in a kitchen several states away.

Also, we rented the house up at Lake George during part of the summer and had no idea what foods other people were bringing into it. At home, I had created a relatively sterilized gluten-free environment. But our renters (not to mention our family, and even us—the former

71

us) had no doubt left a trail of wheat crumbs throughout the kitchen. I worried over things like pots and pans. What if there was a residue of wheat left on the cooking surfaces, the cutting boards, the serving utensils. I would have to pack at least one frying pan and spatula, to be safe, and then guard those items with my life, so that no other family members (the dreaded wheat-eaters, who we shared the house with) would accidentally use them.

My mind leapt to the grill and the tasty hamburgers we were used to indulging in after a long day on the lake. The grill was ancient, and the metal grate had been used for toasting wheat buns for years. I would have to pack tin foil and remind my husband to use it on the grill. Even a speck of gluten could cause contamination.

I started jotting down a list of foods we *could* eat. To be safe, I had to think ahead about every meal and every bite we would eat—not only at Lake George, but while we were on the road.

Okay, I know I'm obsessive. But it's no fun to travel with hungry people. And when you can no longer stop at the nearest convenience store to grab a snack, you have to worry about these things.

Hamburgers. They were a good start. We could eat them at least once or twice, as long as they were grilled on the tin foil or cooked in my clean frying pan. Chicken. Ugh. Thanks to my recent research, I knew that most brands were processed with wheat. I flipped through my handy dandy gluten-free shopping guide and found that there were one or two brands that didn't contain gluten. I would have to either call or look up the grocery stores online to find out if they carried these brands. Just the thought of this made me want to take a very long nap.

Of course, I couldn't help but daydream about the vacations of old (last year!) when we were able to stroll through Lake George Village and pop into any of the local restaurants when we got hungry. I could close my eyes and point to anything on the menu. Nothing was off limits. Our biggest concern was finding something that I liked on the menu. And I say "our" because if I wasn't happy, well, you know the saying, "If Mama ain't happy, ain't nobody happy." Granted, I wasn't that easy to please. But looking back, those days seemed like heaven. Now, we were caught in a gluten-free prison with the not-so-pleasant company of my limited cooking skills.

Packing for our trip was a nightmare for my poor husband. Joel was used to schlepping our numerous bags to the car and spending a good twenty or thirty minutes creating the interlocking puzzle that would allow everything to fit in perfectly.

Now, we had not one, not two, but *three* coolers to add to the car. And I spent hours (or at least it felt like hours) counting eggs, slicing veggies, washing and preparing fruit, freezing meal-sized packs of meat. When my husband would gently ask, "Is this cooler ready to go?" I'd turn on him. "No. Don't touch that! I'm only halfway through my list!" He quickly learned to steer clear of the kitchen until I declared the coolers filled.

The coolers held food for lunches, dinners and snacks, not to mention anything we might want to eat during the next week that I couldn't be sure of finding in a grocery store up north. Once on the road, we would be traveling for sixteen-plus hours, which included a one-night stop at a hotel. During that night, we'd have to bring in our coolers, empty out the melted water and add fresh ice. By the time we reached Lake George, let's just say that most of our food was limp.

Probably the hardest part of those trips was seeing my daughter not be able to participate in certain family activities with the same gusto that the other children did. Sydney and her cousins loved picking blackberries on the family property, returning to our deck and making a sort of blackberry mush out of their ice cream. Blackberries by themselves aren't the same as blackberries and Breyer's.

To our delight, Breyer's Vanilla ice cream was gluten free. But, to our dismay, during that first summer of going gluten free, the villi in Sydney's gut were still healing, so she was only allowed dairy-free ice cream. Besides being hard to find, a frozen-solid concoction made from rice or almond milk certainly didn't look nearly as appealing as the creamy delight everyone else was eating.

I made multiple special trips to the tiny health food store several miles from the lake. The first time I realized it was only open five days a week, and I was there on Monday—you guessed it, one of the days it was closed!

After that I zealously checked the hours and brought the family with me in the hopes that Sydney could pick out some special treats for herself. Joel, Sydney and I spread out, which was hard to do in a store the size of a walk-in closet. We bumped into each other between the frozen section and the bread area.

Sydney pointed to something blue and orange in the freezer. I opened the door and pulled it out, scraping the frost off. The package contained some kind of fruity popsicles. I was about to deposit the box in our shopping basket when I realized I hadn't checked the ingredients. I quickly scanned the label. No gluten. Just red and blue food dye, not to mention high-fructose corn syrup. Great! Let's remove the gluten from Sydney's diet, so we can flood her system with sugar and chemicals.

As I was busy reading the label, Sydney found the candy area. If you could call it candy. There was really nothing recognizable except maybe some sticks of what looked like ancient beef jerky. Sydney pointed to a granola bar in a green wrapper, and Joel—lured by the excitement of a possible sugar high—grabbed a couple. But when he brought them up close to his eyes to read the tiny print on the labels, he started sneezing. I took one and noticed a layer of dust coating my fingers. "How long have these been here? Do you see an expiration date? Are you sure we should get them?"

"No, thanks," said Joel. "I'm going to the regular grocery store."

At that point, Sydney was close to tears. "But I want it."

"Sweetie," I started to explain the dangers of eating spoiled food but thought of the sugar and dyes we were already subjecting her to. I wiped the wrappers across the back of my jeans and threw them in the basket.

Every year, there was a potluck dinner at my cousin Kit's house, and the kids often ate fried chicken or steaming slices of freshly delivered pizza. The table was laden with desserts—cookies, cobblers, cakes, etc.—and none of them were deemed safe. I packed a small green bag with an icepack; a rock-hard, wheat-free muffin; an apple, and our version of pizza—a tasteless gluten-free crust topped with hamburger and rice cheese. (Sydney enjoyed our version until she was brought face-to-face with the real thing.) One of my kind-hearted cousins, who understood the challenges of celiac, made a special effort to bring a gluten-free dessert—brownies—to the family potluck. I could have kissed her! After, that is, I grilled her about the ingredients and made her recite her baking process step-by-step to me. Some people didn't understand, after all, that you couldn't dust a baking pan with regular flour. And I couldn't take the chance. My cousin weathered the inquisition with her typical good humor, and we all enjoyed the brownies.

Still, for Sydney, it was hard to be limited. Always limited. You can have this, but not that. All of those things on the table that the other kids are gobbling up without a thought—the steaming tray of lasagna, the crockpot full of meatballs, the cookies studded with M&Ms, the spice cake with the swirls of vanilla frosting—nope! They might look good. But to you, Sydney, they're poison.

On our way home from the lake, we had to face another long journey. The only thing worse than traveling with three coolers full of food was traveling with three empty coolers. By the end of our vacation, most of our supplies had been eaten or had spoiled. I was either so relaxed after a week at the lake or so focused on getting back home that I adopted Joel's laissez faire attitude about food. I just didn't think through the lengthy trip ahead, nor did I imagine how often we'd get hungry.

I'd managed to shop for and cook all the meals during our seven-day vacation (a first for me). Wasn't that enough? We were planning to make the trip home in one day, so how much food did a family of three need to eat anyway? I had visions of being back in my own kitchen where there was a semi-stocked pantry and a freezer. I could store and defrost food there with ease (at least compared to being on the road).

My feeble attempt at feeding my family on our trip south consisted of cooking some extra hamburgers the night before we left, throwing them in a Tupperware container and making sure we brought the ketchup. Actually, we forgot the ketchup, because who thinks to bring ketchup home when you've been on vacation (if you could call it that) for a week?

So, we ate cold hamburgers for lunch and dinner. I did throw in a half-eaten bag of baby carrots and the remnants of a salad bag for us to snack on. Woo hoo! The bag of salted almonds only went so far. The container of pure maple syrup we had purchased as a special treat for when we got home was looking more and more appealing. Out of desperation, Joel broke down and bought bags of Fritos and tortilla chips from the gas station (after I carefully researched the brand), and we feasted on junk food during the last few hours of the trip.

Joel

*A*fter our trip to Lake George, I got serious about cleaning out our cupboards. The day after Sydney's endoscopy, four months ago, I had gone through the kitchen pitching obvious sources of gluten—boxes of crackers, bags of snacks and packages of cookies, anything that was open and could leave crumbs behind. Some of the food I bagged up and gave to Joel to keep in the back of his car where he could indulge outside the home. Better safe than sorry, I figured.

At least half of what was left in the kitchen had lived there, hiding on back shelves, for years. Not being a cook, I had never really considered what it meant to organize a cabinet, much less a kitchen. So, my spaces were filled with a jumble of canned goods, snack foods, ancient baking ingredients, not to mention odds and ends like a screwdriver, old keys and an occasional piece of junk mail. Don't ask!

My first step was simply to go through everything cabinet by cabinet, shelf by shelf, searching for any and all items that contained gluten. I tossed anything that was outdated and filled grocery bags with food that was still edible to take to the local food pantry or my friend Jean, who had three growing sons and trouble keeping food in the house.

I took the paltry amount of food that was left and arranged it so I'd know what I had. My canned goods had shrunk from one and a half shelves to three cans of gluten-free soup I wasn't sure we'd ever eat.

And instead of a large canister of white flour, I now had a few small plastic bags of strange things like tapioca and almond flours, ingredients the nutritionist had recommended in case I decided to try my hand at cooking from scratch.

Perhaps it was my kitchen clearing fest that inspired Joel to succumb to a gluten-free trial, even though he was certain it wasn't necessary. Sydney and I might be sensitive to gluten, but Joel was used to eating whatever he wanted and was pretty sure his stomach and digestive tract could tolerate anything, including gluten. I figured he was probably right since, compared to me, he had always been the one who was less sensitive—to food, noise, people, anything really. That didn't keep me from occasionally suggesting that he at least *try* going gluten free. After all, celiac ran in families, and he wouldn't know how gluten affected him unless he eliminated it completely from his diet for a period of time.

Joel surprised me one day by announcing he was ready to go off gluten. In fact, without my help, he'd calculated a seven-week trial for himself that would end, auspiciously, on the day he was leaving for a golf trip to the mountains with seven of his guy friends.

As was typical for Joel, once he made a decision, he committed to it. He didn't go back and forth or gnaw on the details as if they were a bone the way I did. Instead, he asked for help in mapping out what was safe for him to eat on a daily basis. I was happy to oblige knowing this could be a step on our journey towards a completely gluten-free household.

Joel's breakfast was usually cereal, and he was happy to eat one of the brands I'd picked up for Sydney at the health food store. Dinners were not a problem because I'd be making those. Lunch was the biggest concern. Joel was now semi-retired, so during the summer, he usually got up early to play golf and came home to eat a sandwich made with whole wheat bread and deli turkey. He'd have to lose the bread, but he seemed fine with the idea of a pile of turkey supplemented with a handful of carrots, an apple and a gluten-free cookie or two.

But if his tee time was midmorning, his old pattern was to buy a hotdog after nine holes at the turn shop or order a late lunch—a BLT, club sandwich or a hamburger with fries—after he finished playing eighteen holes. He could still eat hamburgers and hotdogs, just no buns, and he had to nix the fries in case they were cooked in oil that had been contaminated with gluten.

I took a look at his golf course menu and told him he could have the following sides: a fruit cup, salad or veggies with no toppings. I watched Joel's face to see what his response would be to "no fries." Surprisingly, there was none. He just seemed pleasantly appreciative of my help.

Of course, a small part of me wondered if my husband could really handle gluten-free living. Just because Sydney and I had been doing it for a couple of months didn't mean Joel could cut it. I mean a change like this took intestinal fortitude. No pun intended!

A couple of weeks into his new eating regimen, I asked Joel how it was going. He replied nonchalantly, "Great! It's pretty easy. As long as I know what to eat and what not to eat, I'm fine."

Easy!? He'd forgotten that just the other day I'd grabbed a bag of mixed nuts out of his hands and read the ingredients out loud: "Peanuts, almonds, walnuts, sea salt, wheat!"

"What do you mean wheat? It's a bag of nuts," he said.

"Not all brands are wheat free. You've got to look at the ingredients," I huffed.

He shrugged and looked into the can. "I don't see any wheat. There can't be too much."

"It's enough to hurt Sydney," I said.

"Yeah, maybe. But not me."

Joel's response just underlined how completely different we were. Me—the detail-oriented, slightly neurotic, very protective food planner—vs. him—the relaxed, easygoing, what's-the-problem-with-a-little-wheat guy.

The weeks passed quickly, and every time Sydney and I asked Joel if he felt any different, he'd cock his head as if scanning his body. After a moment's pause, he'd say, "I don't think so. Pretty sure I'm doing this for nothing."

"You might be," I'd respond, "but at least you'll know."

"Yeah, and then I can get back to eating whatever I want," Joel said with a grin.

Over the years, Joel had never been heavy, though his pants had gotten tighter, and he started buying a slightly larger waist size. During the first few weeks of going gluten free, he noticed that his pants were fitting better, and he tightened his belt an extra notch. I complimented him on his flat belly, and he started telling his friends how eating gluten free was a great way to lose weight. I smiled, knowing it wasn't exactly the gluten-free food that was causing the weight loss but the fact that he wasn't snacking as much on whatever happened to be available. Of course, it didn't hurt that he was eating less processed food and more vegetables.

During the last week of Joel's fast from all (or at least *most*) things gluten, I got a phone call from him. He had gone to the nearby town of Salisbury to pick up some golf clubs that had been re-shafted in preparation for his trip to the mountains. He didn't sound like his usual upbeat self.

"Ann, I don't feel so good," he said.

"What's wrong?" I asked. "Are you sick?" It was two days before his trip. Usually he was filled with high energy before a golf trip.

"I feel awful…." His voice was low, and there wasn't a trace of his typical enthusiasm.

"What's going on?" A tiny thought flickered through my mind. Had he fallen off the gluten-free wagon? That couldn't be it. A little gluten had never bothered him before.

Joel unraveled his tale for me. When he went to the golf shop, he found that his clubs weren't quite ready. It was past two o'clock; he'd been on the golf course since early that morning, then on the road to Salisbury, and he was hungry. There was a Subway next door and the scent of fresh-baked bread lured him inside. He quickly rationalized that he was going off gluten in a few days anyway, so why not just grab something.

He ordered one of his old favorites—a six-inch meatball sub—and devoured it quickly. "It's only been twenty minutes, and I feel like I'm hungover," Joel said. "My head's foggy, and I feel rundown. All I want to do is come home and take a nap."

"What?" I'd heard Joel, but I was having trouble computing everything. He'd eaten gluten and done it *before* the deadline he'd given himself. And now he felt awful. Could it be, after all this time, that Joel was just as intolerant to gluten as I was, maybe even Sydney?

"So, you feel bad?" I asked, just to be sure.

"I feel horrible…. I'm never eating wheat again."

Joel having a reaction to gluten was surprising. But Joel making this pronouncement was shocking. I hadn't had to push, pull, encourage or do anything. He figured it out on his own.

Later, I realized that I shouldn't have been so surprised. Anything that would negatively or positively affect Joel's golf game got his attention. Apparently, gluten was bad for golf; going off gluten was good for it. That was all he needed to know. At least for now.

Returning to Fairhaven

*L*ittle did I know, we would return to Fairhaven over and over after Sydney's diagnosis. The staff remembered us after we'd sent them a loaf of bread for the ducks, along with this note from Sydney: "Please tell the duckies I haven't forgotten them. And give them this bread. Thank you." They had responded with a letter to Sydney saying they'd be sure to feed them throughout the year and that the ducks would be waiting for her when she returned. We promised Sydney we'd drive back to the mountains during the fall break of her Kindergarten. Once again, we spent three days and two nights.

Fairhaven became a place of transition, a spot where our family could vacation and rest and learn to weave in gluten-free cooking without the whole ordeal thoroughly exhausting me.

There were losses such as the delicious chocolate chip cookies made with wheat. When we returned to Fairhaven, as soon as we walked into our chalet, I moved the cookie jar to the top of the refrigerator, so it would be out of sight. Fortunately, I had planned ahead and made our own gluten-free cookies in advance, so we'd have some treats after our meals.

Going out to dinner like we had in the past wasn't so hard to give up because we didn't really want to leave Fairhaven anyway. The quiet beauty of the mountains, the ducks, the trails, the games and the books were enough to keep our family of three entertained.

It might have been nice to have some food delivered. But knowing that wasn't an option, it seemed "worth it" to cook our meals in the little kitchen. Yes, I had to pack a lot of food—not just the easy breakfast and lunch items (eggs, cereal, milk, bread and deli turkey), but meat for our main dishes, vegetables, snacks, cooking oil, spices, ketchup, butter, a clean cutting board—everything and anything we might need.

But there were clean pots, pans, dishes and utensils at the chalet. There was also the bonus of eating outside on the front deck and games like croquet to distract us. And I had peace of mind knowing I could feed our family safely. For Joel, the worst part was having to do the dishes when there was no dishwasher. (It was only fair that I cooked, and he cleaned.) But even he settled into our new gluten-free rhythm without complaint.

I realized later that feeding the ducks and handling wheat bread three times a day (the ducks needed breakfast, lunch and dinner just like us, according to Sydney) during that first trip to Fairhaven had probably exacerbated her symptoms of bloating, constipation and sleeplessness. But after her celiac diagnosis, we brought a loaf of gluten-free bread with us. It cost four times the amount of regular bread, so Sydney could have just as easily been throwing quarters to the ducks. But it was worth it knowing our daughter wasn't constantly touching wheat.

Attitude

When you're raising a child to be gluten free, you have to adopt an attitude. Your daughter, who has never lived with any food restrictions, suddenly has over fifty percent of the things she used to enjoy taken away from her. What do you say? How do you make this a good thing? Is it a good thing?

"Honey, we are so fortunate that you have celiac, because now we can all eat a healthier diet." "Sweetie, I know it's hard. But think how good you feel." "You have changed our lives for the better. We're all going to live to be one hundred and ten now." Of course, who cares how long we live, if we can't treat ourselves?

It was true. We were all eating more healthfully. I discovered that vegetables really were a food group. Both Joel and I lost a few pounds. As I weaned myself from gluten, I realized that I felt better. I had less bloating, fewer headaches, I slept better, and any mild depression I had seemed to evaporate.

But I still missed cookies. After all, I had a long-standing relationship with the chocolate chip variety. Once I started obsessing over them, anything could happen. These cookies were my friends. I couldn't just abandon them, could I? It wasn't like I had celiac. Or at least no blood test had confirmed it. Maybe all this concern about gluten was in my head. Yes, there were gluten-free cookies that satisfied me most of the time, but every once in a while, I just felt like I needed the real thing. What could it hurt? Just one.

The cookie tasted awfully good going down—the tender, crumbly sweetness—there was no way it would affect me. For the first ten minutes, I felt smug. See, I can eat wheat. What a lot of bother this has been. All this gluten-free hubbub over nothing.

But gradually, I felt a tiredness creeping over me. And my brain slowed down as if a low fog bank had rolled in. An hour or so later, my digestive tract became sluggish, and I felt bloated. It was as if there was a drag on my whole body, along with a weird sensation in my limbs and joints. That night, I was restless and awake at 2 a.m., frustrated by my insomnia and aware on a gut level (literally!) that my body and gluten were not compatible.

I slipped off the gluten-free wagon a couple more times. Usually it happened during a moment of weakness, when I was sad about my mother's Alzheimer's or tired from caretaking or missing too much sleep. The desire for comfort was stronger than the memory of what it felt like to have gluten enter my body, so I would succumb. But each cookie indulgence made a deeper impression on me. I didn't want to feel bad. Cookies filled with gluten made everything worse.

Finally, something in my mind clicked. I didn't have to eat them. There were other ways I could treat myself. Eating gluten wasn't worth feeling rotten for a few days. It was as if a metal gate clanged shut inside me, leaving cookies made with wheat on the outside. I was actually really, really happy to be done with them, and I never wanted to let wheat or any of its gluten-y cousins into my body again.

Sydney couldn't experiment like I could. Gluten was her sworn enemy. We didn't actually know what would happen if she had an exposure, now that she'd been off of gluten for several months. She had thrown up the first time, when Joel had taken her to the store, and they'd eaten food that wasn't gluten free off the sample table. It was likely her reaction would be stronger now. No matter what, though, we knew that wheat would cause damage to her intestines.

Sydney hardly remembered a time when her stomach hurt, even though it wasn't so long ago. She was young. She didn't care that she grew several inches the summer after she got off gluten. What she cared about was that she couldn't eat what her friends were eating. She didn't want to be different. And who could blame her? It's no fun to be the only one at a party who can't eat the cake, to not be able to join in on cookie baking, gingerbread house making, dessert trolling at potluck meals. I never realized how many activities revolved around food until my daughter couldn't participate.

At the same time, I didn't want Sydney to think that her life was miserable or that she was a victim. I mean, come on. We happened to live in one of the richest countries in the world, and yet, she couldn't have everything that all the other kids could have. But she was certainly not starving. She lived a privileged life. We were fortunate to be able to afford gluten-free food. And for gosh sakes, she had a mom who ran around providing her gluten-free alternatives every time there was a birthday party.

It was a fine line to walk—trying to help Sydney be aware that her celiac was a mixed blessing. We were healthier for it. Yes, it was painful to be left out. I tried to emphasize that everyone had something challenging in their life, even if she couldn't see it. The neighbor down the street had lost his dog. One of her best friends was adopted and would likely never know her birth mother. The boy in her class, who could eat whatever he wanted, had a family that had been split by divorce. Some people have to live with physical pain, and some endure emotional pain. Most eventually learn to deal with some degree of both.

In the end, I had to trust that God had given Sydney this condition and he would care for her. We, as a family, would learn to cope. And so would she.

School

*B*efore getting acquainted with celiac disease, I wouldn't have thought food allergies would have much, if any, bearing on where Sydney went to school. I mean school is supposed to be about academics, quality teachers, the right community, a good athletic program. Not lunch. Right?

Sydney was diagnosed at the age of five, during the spring of her last year of preschool. We were fortunate to have wonderful, kind and caring teachers who took a real interest in our daughter's condition. One of them even invited Sydney to share her endoscopy photos during Show & Tell.

But snack time with a room full of four and five-year-olds was not the ideal setting for a newly diagnosed celiac patient. Little hands and crumbs everywhere! Can you say cross-contamination?

It was also hard for Sydney to suddenly not be allowed to eat the goldfish she had enjoyed all year, not to mention watching her classmates continue to gobble them every morning without a thought. Even the fruit juices served in little cups along with the snacks had to be examined thoroughly for "added flavors." With some research I was able to find a couple of brands of safe, gluten-free juice, and every morning I stopped by the local health food store to prowl the aisles for gluten-free goodies that might hold as much allure as the banned goldfish.

In the early days after Sydney's celiac diagnosis, we fell into a new pattern. Every day, after picking her up from preschool, she'd ask me what I found at the store. I'd produce an array of gluten-free items for her to try in hopes of finding palatable substitutes for the snacks she'd given up. There were crackers that usually tasted like cardboard, frozen bagels, granola bars, cookies. Her favorite treat ended up being Annie's Bunnies, probably because they were shaped like little rabbits and similar in size to the goldfish. She also liked fruit, raisins and gluten-free pretzel sticks, which tasted surprisingly like the regular, gluten-filled ones.

Even at the age of five, Sydney was wise and careful enough to stay away from what her friends were eating. And because her snacks were different, many of the kids asked if they could share *her* food. Her friends insisted that the gluten-free pretzels were better than the traditional ones. I would have been happy to supply the entire class with gluten-free snacks through the end of the year, except for the fact that they cost three times as much for less than half the amount.

By the end of preschool, Joel and I had already had many discussions about where Sydney would go to Kindergarten. We had toured several of the local schools. Once we began to understand the challenges we were facing with shifting to a gluten-free diet and the importance of strict adherence for Sydney's health, our choices suddenly narrowed to schools that were in easy driving distance. I wanted to be close enough that I could run over and deliver snacks or a birthday treat.

We ended up choosing a private school that was literally around the corner from us. Both Joel and I were products of public school, but I wasn't ready to face gluten on such a large scale. And we were fortunate we could afford private education. I assumed a small school would make things easier. I knew I'd have to meet with her future teacher to impress upon her the importance and details of our daughter's diet. Along with wanting to keep Sydney healthy and feeling good, I hoped to be able to share the emotional side of the situation. While I trusted Sydney to know what she could and couldn't eat, I didn't want her to always be on the outside looking in. Like any child, she wanted to participate and eat what the other kids were eating.

We hit the jackpot with Sydney's teachers—Mrs. Maynor, who was young, sweet and eager to please, and her kind-hearted assistant. They listened carefully as I explained how even a small amount of gluten could set off a reaction in Sydney. They assured me they would do everything in their power to not only keep Sydney safe, but help her feel included.

The only problem was that the school was closed—literally locked—for security reasons during the day. Parents had to have special permission to enter the building. I had envisioned being able to walk Sydney to her classroom, check in with the teacher, peek in the classroom and have a direct line of communication. But no. Parents dropped their kids off in the carpool line. We would say our goodbyes in the car, and I'd watch my daughter disappear behind the big metal doors of school, a place I imagined was crawling with gluten.

I would have to become a sleuth to find out just what was going on behind those closed doors. Thankfully, at the beginning of the year, Mrs. Maynor invited me to be a Room Mother, so I could attend all of the special class functions. I took advantage of every opportunity, so I could see for myself what the gluten situation was like at school. I signed up for Fun Fridays where I could visit Sydney's classroom for an hour once a month and read to the students or do an activity. The school had a weekly chapel service that was open to parents, and I got to know the cafeteria staff and the librarian.

Sydney's birthday was early in the school year and happened to be the same day as the class's first field trip. Parents were allowed to bring treats and join in on birthday celebrations. So, I went along to the animal park and brought a cooler full of gluten-free snacks and juice. I picked up a tray of regular cupcakes at the grocery store and ordered half a dozen specially made gluten-free cupcakes from a bakery and asked them to match the color and design of the store-bought ones. It was a dream for Sydney to be able to eat something that looked like what everyone else was eating.

I gave Mrs. Maynor my phone number and offered to bring gluten-free treats to school any time she planned an event that involved food.

Mrs. Maynor was thoughtful and conscientious about calling me. Sometimes it was at the last minute, but knowing how busy her day was, I so appreciated her efforts to keep me informed and thanked her profusely. Her sensitivity to the situation was heartwarming.

But I learned from Sydney that special occasions involving food at the school were not occasional. Other than recognized holidays, it was impossible to plan around them. Gluten was everywhere. Teachers and staff handed out candy and food on an almost daily basis—during assemblies, on the playground, during chapel and lunch.

I supplied Mrs. Maynor with a bag of gluten-free candy and snacks to keep in the classroom and stored a box of frozen gluten-free donuts and frosted muffins in the cafeteria, in hopes that Sydney wouldn't be left out during impromptu celebrations. I even printed out a list of gluten-free foods for all the parents. But, despite my vigilance, parents inevitably (and understandably) brought birthday or holiday treats into the classroom that Sydney couldn't eat. Yes, she could retrieve something from her gluten-free stash, but it never quite lived up to the sugary delights the other kids were indulging in. Who would choose a rock-hard muffin from the freezer over a slice of cake decorated with Disney characters or freshly baked Christmas cookies smothered with icing and sprinkles? My heart broke a little each time Sydney came home from school and told me how her classmates all got a special treat. But there wasn't anything for her. It didn't happen every day. But it happened a lot.

Friends

*M*ost of our family and friends continued to eat the way they normally did. In front of us. They ordered plates overflowing with gluten delicacies—hamburgers with fluffy gluten rolls, French fries sautéed up in cross-contaminated oil, ketchup with modified starch (yikes!), chicken processed with wheat and grilled on a gluteny grill, pasta made of curly bits of gluten, sauces thickened with flour...I mean gluten. And those were the things that didn't bother us.

It was when the three-layer cakes filled with blueberry preserves, the chocolate fudge, the homemade cupcakes and brownies, the trays and trays of every imaginable cookie lined the tables and counters, and our friends dug into their dessert plates, as every good red-blooded American does, that we began to feel deprived. I said "we," but I really meant Sydney, because I turned my nose up and pretended those desserts didn't exist, while Joel, at least in the beginning, wasn't able to stop himself from indulging, even if he did feel awful an hour later.

Our family was suddenly on the wrong side of the fence, outside of a world we had once been a part of and thoroughly enjoyed. Now, we watched as a parade of our favorite foods marched just under our drooling lips on a regular basis.

Of course, as Sydney's mother, I tried to interest her in something else. "Oh, look at this beautiful apple! Doesn't it look delicious?" And when that didn't work, I'd suggest in a slightly superior way that *those* people had no idea what they were putting into their bodies, and that one day they'd regret it.

Sydney didn't fall for any of it. She knew she was getting a raw deal, and she wasn't happy about it.

So, when a few beloved friends took note of our desperate situation and made the effort to bake something gluten free for us, we did our version of the happy dance. I nervously asked about every single ingredient (Do you mind if I take a peek at the box or package this dessert came from?) and tried to ferret out whether they had used a pan that might have a residue of gluten on it. When deemed "safe," Sydney and Joel would have not one, not two, but three servings, just in case the delicacy might vanish when they weren't looking.

When friends put up with my "gluten anxiety," my never-ending questions and *still* wanted to bake treats for our family, and did it happily, generously and lovingly, I was truly overwhelmed with gratitude.

We've experienced friends all along the spectrum—those who belonged in heaven with a glowing halo because of their incredible awareness and compassion and others who didn't have a clue that the moisture on the table was saliva dripping down our chins as we watched them devour their dinners. Even though it was frustrating at times, I could never get too upset with those who appeared to be blind to gluten. After all, I had been one of them not so long ago.

I still remembered offering a slice of my egg casserole to my friend Gilda, not once, but numerous times, after she'd told me repeatedly that she reacted badly to wheat and gluten. "It only has a *little* bit of gluten in it," I wheedled, clearly more interested in the kudos I hoped to receive because I'd actually cooked something, than her health and comfort.

The casserole was made of eggs, milk, cheese, broccoli, squash and torn up pieces of bread. Bread made from wheat! At that time, I had no clue that there was even such a thing as gluten-free bread. Nor did I imagine that small bits of it could affect anyone in such a dire way as to cause major intestinal distress, let alone severe inflammation. And I considered myself a good and caring friend.

So, it was easy for me to give a pass to those who didn't understand, even those who looked askance at me when I spent an extra ten minutes questioning the waiter about food preparation or pulled my own baggie or thermos of safely prepared chicken out of my personal bag lined with cold packs.

Sadly, I couldn't name even one person who had an allergy when I was growing up. No doubt a few of these folks existed, even if celiac was rarely diagnosed back then. But I most likely simply dismissed them. Without thinking, I slid an imaginary curtain between them and me. I didn't understand what they were going through, so it wasn't my concern. I cringe now at how selfish I was.

If there's such a thing as karma, I'm receiving mine in spades. Of course, allergies are much more prevalent these days, and kids with food sensitivities seem to find each other. Sydney has friends with gluten, dairy, corn, soy and many more allergies. So, I've had plenty of opportunities to change my ways.

Homeschool

$\mathcal{A}$ s I look back, it doesn't surprise me that when the opportunity to homeschool Sydney arose, we took it. My mother passed away during the fall when Sydney was in Kindergarten, and her school closed unexpectedly the following May. Joel and I jumped into action researching and touring all the local private schools. We considered public school, but with Sydney's celiac disease I was most concerned about keeping her healthy. Public schools had larger classes and basically what seemed to be more opportunities for gluten exposures.

We enrolled Sydney in a Montessori school for first grade. It was only a mile or two further away from our home than her other school. I liked the diversity of students and the relaxed environment. Parents were welcome to visit any time, and, in fact, were called on to help with certain events or drive students to off-campus activities.

I packed Sydney's lunch each day as I'd done in Kindergarten, provided a bag of gluten-free snacks and sweets for the teacher to keep in the classroom and created a suggested list of gluten-free items for the other parents to bring during special events.

Sydney still reported incidents where her classmates received gluten-filled treats while she looked on longingly. But we were both more used to this kind of thing, and I realized that, sadly, it was inevitable. We simply couldn't expect everyone else to understand the danger that gluten posed to those with celiac, nor could we hold them responsible for making sure Sydney didn't feel left out.

However, a couple of families stood out that year. Sydney became friends with Ellie and Natalie, two sisters who had been adopted. I got to know their mother who worked at the front desk of the school. On sunny afternoons after school, Joanne and I would sit on a bench by the garden and talk as our girls played together. Over time, I shared about our gluten-free journey. We took the girls on playdates, and Joanne always made a special effort to provide gluten-free snacks for Sydney.

During that same year, Sydney also got to know a sweet girl named Maia, and Joel and I became close with her parents—Charles and Samantha—as we attended various school events.

Our three families ended up making the decision to homeschool the next year. Each of us had different reasons, but our bonds grew deeper as we shared this journey. Joanne, Samantha and I got the girls together regularly, and they attended various activities and classes as a group.

For me, when it came to avoiding gluten, homeschool was a relief. Sydney ate most of her meals and snacks at home. Fear of a gluten contamination vanished, and gluten-filled treats were no longer paraded under Sydney's nose on an almost daily basis. Sydney's celiac disease became a nonissue. Because everyone in our family avoided gluten, it became the norm to eat the way we did. We were only confronted with the Standard American Diet when we went out or gathered with large groups of other homeschoolers.

Most often, we socialized with a small group of kids and moms that we got to know well. It wasn't unusual for everyone to bring a bagged lunch to outings. If we did go to a restaurant, our friends would ask where Sydney and I could eat.

A handful of other homeschoolers that we met during that time also had allergies. I was actually surprised how many families had unique reasons for homeschooling. They ranged from learning disabilities to health issues to academic concerns to convenience. Having a condition that required a gluten-free diet seemed insignificant compared to the issues with which many other parents and families were dealing.

In many ways, we were spoiled because we had such kind friends and a wonderful community. It was great fun to gather with them, meet at the park or host an activity at our house. The other moms were always thoughtful. Sometimes I had to remind them that Sydney was gluten free. But once I clued them in, they wanted to know more, and they always made an effort to make sure Sydney felt included.

I have so many special memories from those years. For example, I'll never forget how Samantha invited the girls and moms to join her and Maia for a cooking date at their house. She bought them all matching aprons and provided gluten-free ingredients so that Sydney, Maia, Ellie and Natalie could all make the same kind of cookies. Sydney could lick the spoon or sample the batter just like the others. There was much laughter and joy in Samantha's kitchen that day, and my heart overflowed with appreciation.

After we'd been homeschooling for about a year and a half, Sydney met Lauren-Kate in a sewing class. Sydney's close friends Ellie and Natalie had recently moved to Texas, and Lauren-Kate was in the process of saying goodbye to good friends who were also moving away. Lauren-Kate's mom Karen and I arranged a playdate for our daughters.

Karen and I were surprised to learn all the similarities between the girls. Sydney was an only child, while Lauren-Kate was the only child still at home. Sydney had celiac disease and Lauren-Kate was "allergic" to gluten. Both girls were also homeschooled, nature lovers and crazy about animals. Each of them even had a cat they adored. With their fair skin and blond hair, they were often mistaken for sisters (as were Karen and I). We even discovered that we both had family in upstate New York in towns less than an hour apart.

The girls enjoyed spending time together, and Karen and I became good friends. We lived within ten minutes of each other, so we got the girls together for frequent playdates over the summer. While the girls played, Karen and I talked. We were both interested in homeschool, parenting and health topics and could talk endlessly on any of these subjects.

Karen wasn't quite as vigilant about gluten as I was because Lauren-Kate hadn't been officially diagnosed with celiac, but she understood my concerns and was well aware of the dangers. One of Lauren-Kate's friends who had moved away actually had celiac, and Karen was used to cooking for her. Because of the similarity in the girls' diets (and Karen's awareness about gluten), it was easy to drop Sydney off at their house or have Lauren-Kate spend the day with us. The girls would spend hours outside at Karen's house or down by the creek in front of ours. For snacks, Karen or I would cut up apples and provide rolls of turkey or gluten-free crackers. We didn't have to play detective with each other to find out what might be lurking in our kitchens. Karen and I were on the same page when it came to preparing healthy food for our girls.

It didn't take long before we arranged for the girls to take classes together. For four years, I taught a writing class for them. Sydney and Lauren-Kate attended various other activities together such as an art class, a physical education class, programs at our local park, even Science Olympiad.

Karen organized a mother/daughter book club at her house that we joined for several years. Four moms with five daughters gathered monthly, and Karen, who loved to cook, always provided gluten-free snacks for the girls. This sweet group of girls discussed books, played together and sat around the table eating snacks, and I was so grateful for this community where food had become a nonissue.

Caspian

When Sydney was first diagnosed with celiac disease, I had no idea what the ripple effect would be. What I did know was that I felt the need to share our story with everyone and anyone who would listen. Our lives had changed, were changing in unexpected, indescribable ways. We were undergoing a transformation that I hadn't known (years ago) that I needed and didn't realize until now was even possible.

I wanted others to know about the dangers of gluten. It wasn't just responsible for typical symptoms such as fatigue, digestive complaints, nausea or weight loss. From my reading and research, I picked up that there were many conditions such as diabetes, irritable bowel syndrome, migraines, liver disease, epilepsy, Down's Syndrome and Sjogren's disease, to name a few, associated with people who had celiac and gluten intolerance. While doctors were reluctant to draw a direct link (due to the lack of testing and studies), I couldn't help but have my suspicions.

When friends or family brought up physical symptoms they were experiencing, I would often go silent for a moment. Then I'd clear my throat and say slowly, "You know there's a chance that gluten could be involved."

In my mind, gluten had become the culprit (or at least a likely suspect) in a wide variety of ailments. Online sites had lists of symptoms of gluten intolerance that encompassed issues like depression, psoriasis or itchy skin, infertility, weight gain, discoloration of teeth, intestinal cancer, thyroid disease and so on.

I witnessed the transformation Sydney was undergoing on a gluten-free diet, and I experienced my own health revival. How could I not believe that what people put into their bodies affected them? With an intolerance to gluten and the fact that the Standard American Diet included wheat in every meal, was it really surprising that people's cells were not being properly nourished but instead were, in a variety of ways, metaphorically screaming?

That's not to say that everyone agreed with me, or even that I swallowed all of my own theories lock, stock and barrel. I wasn't one to proselytize. But I listened and offered my alternative opinions to anyone who might be open to them.

I met Megan in our church nursery a few years after Sydney's diagnosis. Megan was a young mom, pretty and vivacious. But that morning, she had circles under her eyes. She told me she was exhausted because her baby had been keeping her up night after night. My heart went out to her as I vividly recalled the anguish of my own sleepless nights. A tiny bell went off in my head. But lots of babies have trouble sleeping, I told myself. Besides, I had just met her. I didn't want to overwhelm her with my theories on gluten.

During our chat, I learned that Megan's mom had had early-onset Alzheimer's. As a high school student Megan cared for her mom, coming home at lunchtime to feed her each day. I felt an instant bond with her because of my own mother's illness. And the tiny bell sounded again. Louder this time.

A few weeks later, Megan and I both attended a women's breakfast at my friend Jean's house. Jean had helped me come up with my first list of gluten-free meals. In her kitchen, we sat around the table and shared bits and pieces of our lives with the other women from our church. I learned more about Megan as she talked of being trained as a nurse and how she enjoyed scoping out garage sales on Saturday mornings for great deals. She loved gardening, and she and her husband Mitch wanted to have more children. But there was a weariness in her eyes that I recognized. Her son was still not sleeping through the night.

Celiac presents differently in different people, but if there was any chance I could save Megan from some of the difficulties I had gone through, I wanted to do it. After breakfast, most of the women moved into Jean's living room. This gave me an opportunity to talk with Megan in the kitchen privately

I asked questions and told her Sydney's story. Megan's son Caspian, like Sydney, was small for his age. She told me he barely registered on the growth chart. He didn't just wake up in the middle of the night. He hardly napped and didn't come close to the twelve-plus hours of sleep recommended for a one-year-old baby.

"What's his diet like?" The questions came fast to my mind. "Does his stomach ever hurt?"

I didn't want to barge in with all the answers. Of course, I had no proof of anything. But the similarities between Caspian and Sydney when she was a baby were uncanny. With everything I was hearing from Megan, I told her there was enough evidence that I thought it was worth getting Caspian checked for celiac.

Megan listened intently and took my suggestion seriously.

A few weeks later, I saw her at church, and she told me she'd had Caspian tested. To my surprise (but not shock), the tests showed that Caspian had celiac. She was incredibly relieved and thankful to know what the problem was, but with her background in nursing, she bemoaned the fact that she hadn't known sooner. I quickly told her what I had recently read—that most people who have celiac don't get a diagnosis for at least eleven years after their symptoms begin showing, so she was way ahead of the curve.

Megan and I continued to talk weekly on Sunday mornings, catching up on each other's lives and sharing information about gluten-free resources. Megan took the same kind of extreme care with Caspian's diet that I did with Sydney's. Maybe even more. In the nursery, he was the only child with a "green" smoothie in his sippy cup. She and Caspian have been rewarded with results—better sleep, more growth and all-around improved health.

The next summer, when Sydney was eight, Megan asked if she would like to be a Mother's Helper. Megan looked forward to having a couple of hours to work on her own projects each week, and she knew how important it was for her son to be around someone else who couldn't have gluten. Sydney had always loved children and spending time with Caspian was a treat for her. As for me, I enjoyed being able to check in on my sweet friend. Megan and I usually spent a few minutes talking about health issues, gluten-free recipes or life when I dropped Sydney off or picked her up.

Now, eight years later, Megan and her husband have four children. Sydney has been Megan's primary babysitter throughout this period of time, even despite several local moves. Caspian is the only child with confirmed celiac disease in the family, though Megan was also recently diagnosed, and her home is generally gluten-free. Sydney, who always yearned for siblings, has literally watched Caspian grow up, and she has embraced all of Megan's kids. I never could have dreamed that celiac would bring the gift of these kinds of special connections.

Summer Camp

$\mathcal{F}$ or most families, summer camp is something to look forward to—
an escape from the routine, an opportunity for kids to meet new
friends and have new experiences, a chance for them to develop a sense
of independence, a window of time for parents to be kids again. After
all, the kids at summer camp will be looked after; they'll be surrounded
by other children; their days and activities will be scheduled, and
there's tons of fun on the agenda. What could be better?

Sydney was only nine when she went away to her first summer
camp. It was hard to explain to other parents why I had misgivings. It
wasn't her age or her temperament. From practically the moment she
was born, Sydney loved being with other kids. As she grew older, the
more people that were in the house, the happier Sydney was. And
everything was great, as long as we were in our house where I could
control food and snacks and barricade the door against the uninvited
guest—gluten.

Now that Sydney's system had been virtually cleared of gluten, we
had no idea what an exposure would do to her. As an allergen, gluten
hadn't received the acclaim that peanuts had. It wouldn't cause my
daughter to go into anaphylactic shock. But it would most likely cause
her to feel sick and nauseous. As with the nutritionist's daughter, she
might retch over and over until every speck of gluten was eliminated
from her body. Not to mention that even the smallest amount of wheat

could cause stomach pain, lack of energy and an inability to sleep—none of which would make for a pleasant summer camp experience.

There were a handful of camps (there are more these days) that offered allergen-free menus, groups of kids that experienced camp life with a sterile kitchen environment and the company of others who suffered from similar conditions.

But this was real life. And Sydney wanted to go to a "normal" camp—the one that her friends from church were attending. I'd heard wonderful things about this camp. The counselors were awesome; the other kids were great; the games, the songs, the lake activities were all highly touted.

But the kitchen was a gluten minefield. It would be hard to serve a couple hundred campers who eat gluten for every meal and keep my daughter—the one and only child with celiac—safe.

We had a few things going for us. One was that Sydney was not so sensitive to gluten that she'd get sick if she touched it—as long as she wasn't handling it all day long or living in a cloud of wheat flour. However, it would likely only take a crumb to make her ill. But she'd have to ingest that crumb. Not breathe it or brush against it.

The second thing was that Penny, the mom of one of Sydney's friends, would be working in the kitchen. We had multiple conversations where she encouraged me to allow Sydney to attend camp. Penny and her daughter Lizzie told us all about the bunkhouses, what mealtimes were like and the various activities the kids loved. She assured me that she would do everything she could to keep Sydney safe.

Sydney, of course, wondered why I couldn't go to camp with her and work in the kitchen like Lizzie's mom. A part of me would have done that in a heartbeat—the part of me that would do anything and everything to keep my sweet girl safe. Unfortunately, there was also a part of me that was an exhausted, introverted noncook. The thought of being surrounded by a camp full of kids all day, every day could send me over the edge. Still, I looked into it. Maybe I could help out at mealtimes and then find a quiet place to retreat. Perhaps it was providence that the camp only accepted a certain number of kitchen helpers, and they had reached their limit that summer. Apparently, Sydney was not the only child who wanted her mom close by.

I told Sydney I could not be at camp, but I would do the next best thing. I would prepare a cooler of all her favorite foods and meals that she could eat. That seemed to satisfy her.

"Don't forget the Ranch House!" she reminded me, before running off to play. The Ranch House was the place where kids lined up each afternoon at camp to buy snacks and cold drinks. It was a tradition she wanted to experience.

What had I gotten myself into? I didn't have time to worry about it for long. Camp would be starting a week after we returned home from our vacation at Lake George.

I'd have one week to prepare enough breakfasts, lunches, dinners and snacks to get her through five and a half days of camp. One week! Did I mention that I'm not a cook? How about the fact that we'd just be getting home from several days of being out of town, days where I'd already taken on the responsibility of preparing every meal after shopping at unfamiliar grocery stores. We'd made the trip to Lake George for a few years in a row now, and I had a routine down. But, still, it wasn't easy! At least I had a week.

The first thing I did was contact the camp director to let him know about Sydney's celiac disease. I asked him to put me in touch with the head cook. The staff was kind and eager to accommodate me. Yes, the cook was familiar with celiac. They'd had kids who had allergies at the camp before. But, unfortunately, Sydney was the only one he knew of with celiac during her camp session. He seemed relieved to hear that I would provide food for her. I asked for a copy of a typical week's menu, and he told me what they sold at the Ranch House. None of it sounded safe. But he said I could pack a box of snacks for Sydney, and they would keep it in the Ranch House. That way she could stand in line like the other kids and ask for something out of her box.

Once the cook emailed me the camp menu, I studied it carefully to see which meals I could replicate with gluten-free food. Then I typed up my own camp menu filling in reasonable substitutes. For example, in place of Chicken Alfredo, I inserted our own version of Creamy Chicken and Broccoli. Spaghetti would have to do for lasagna. I couldn't even trust the camp hamburgers. They might be cooked on a surface contaminated by crumbs from the wheat-filled buns.

I made sure Sydney okayed each substitution because if she didn't like the meal, she'd be out of luck. She couldn't just ask the cook to bring her something different. Even the junk food that every camper typically fills up on would not be safe for her.

After getting home from Lake George, I set up shop in the kitchen. I would be cooking and baking more than I'd ever cooked and baked in my life. I told Joel and Sydney that I was UNAVAILABLE the week before camp. Except for last-minute runs to Target for camp items or quick trips to the health food store, I would be sequestered in the kitchen. Joel and Sydney were wise enough to leave me alone most of the time because they could tell my stress level was high.

For every breakfast, lunch and dinner meal that week before camp, I made double the amount of food I normally would, then labelled and froze half of it. The labels noted the day of the week, which meal, what type of food it was and how long to heat it, along with Sydney's name. To make it simple for the kitchen staff, I placed everything for one meal inside of a large clear bag and labeled it, so that it would be easy to simply pull out "Monday's breakfast" or "Tuesday's dinner." I made copies of my own version of the Camp Menu and put them inside sheet protectors—one for the head cook and another securely taped on top of the cooler, so that it would be relatively effortless for anyone to match the food to the correct meal.

We spent a fortune on extras that Sydney didn't usually eat like gluten-free buns, graham crackers, chocolate bars and marshmallows that were safe, so that she could join in the typical camp activities like cookouts and making s'mores. I labelled several plastic baggies of s'mores ingredients and placed them in a brown paper bag filled with chips and other dry snacks. I made sure to write Sydney's name and what was in each bag on the outside in big letters.

Because camp is a veritable sugar fest, and I didn't want Sydney to be left out of the fun, I made sure she had desserts for every meal, including things like homemade cookies for the Cookie Mush, a special night where the kids were served a dessert made of layers of chilled whipped topping, cookie crumbs and milk.

The ice cream was a little trickier. Most people didn't realize that regular ice cream often had gluten in it. In fact, after my research, I only discovered two brands that were gluten-free—Edy's and Breyer's—and not every flavor was safe. The camp most likely purchased bulk containers of ice cream, and any kitchen staff who didn't understand celiac might serve up a dish to Sydney. We would have to provide a carton of ice cream that would be safe for her to eat. Unfortunately, there was no way I could send frozen ice cream on a two-hour bus ride and expect it to be anything other than soup upon arrival.

So, Joel and I made a plan. We'd ask the camp moms to deliver our large cooler to the kitchen on the first day of camp. Joel and I would drive up to the mountains the next day, pick up a carton of gluten-free vanilla ice cream and drop it off at camp for her, along with a box of snacks, water bottles and drinks for the Ranch House. If we timed it right, we might even get a short visit with Sydney before lunch.

We could have given the name and brand of the ice cream to the head cook and asked him to buy it. But what if it wasn't available? The two brands of ice cream that offered gluten-free flavors didn't label their product "gluten free." You had to be willing to read through the long list of ingredients in tiny print and be aware of words like "barley malt" or even "artificial flavors." Unless you were a certified gluten detective (like me), it would be easy to miss something, and I didn't want to risk Sydney's health, especially during the first week our daughter would be away at camp. Not to mention the fact that ice cream was important to Sydney. It was one of the few desserts that she loved and could enjoy along with her friends. It would have broken her heart (and mine!) for her to have to watch the other campers indulge in this special treat and not be able to join them.

Lest anyone get the wrong idea, the trip to the mountains wasn't all about Sydney. Joel and I had planned a long-awaited visit to a special mountain hideaway in Blowing Rock, a couple of hours from camp. It was rare for us to take a trip together, just the two of us. In fact, other than celebrating an occasional anniversary by spending a night in a local hotel, we just didn't go anywhere together. With my mother's Alzheimer's and my in-laws living some distance away, we didn't have grandparents who could step in and help with childcare. So, to say I was looking forward to this trip was an understatement. Of course, with all the cooking I'd been doing, I envisioned getting to Blowing Rock, walking to the bedroom, crawling under the covers and sleeping for three straight days.

The morning before camp started, Joel and I drove into Charlotte where three buses would pick up the campers and drive to the foothills of Western North Carolina. Some parents chose to take their kids to camp in their own cars, but the bus trip was part of the fun, according to Sydney's friend Lizzie, and neither of them wanted to miss out.

We rendezvoused with Penny and another mom who would be working in the kitchen and gave them our cooler and several bags of food. Penny assured me she'd keep an eye on things and let us know if Sydney had any problems. Still, my heart twisted in my chest as I hugged Sydney goodbye and she boarded the bus. Joel and I waved to her through the window.

While we waited for the bus to leave, the driver opened the door to allow parents to come inside and take photos. I couldn't resist the opportunity to climb on, give Sydney another quick hug and snap a photo of her and Lizzie. They were both beaming—smiling and laughing as they prepared for their big adventure. The joy on their sweet faces gave me peace.

Our first night at home without Sydney felt strange and, frankly, just plain wrong. My radar hadn't adjusted to not having a child in the house.

At first, every time I walked by Sydney's room or thought of our sweet girl, I imagined that she was in the safe circumference of our home. It was a shock to my system when I remembered that she was miles away at camp! But whenever I felt a twinge of anxiety, I pulled up the last photo I had taken of Sydney's glowing face. I knew she would miss us. But she loved being with friends. I said a quick prayer that she would have fun and that food would not be an issue.

The next day, Joel and I drove to the mountains, stopped by the grocery store near the camp and picked up a half gallon of gluten-free vanilla ice cream. It was almost noon as we drove down the long road to the camp. Perfect timing! We could meet the cook, drop off the ice cream, visit with Lizzie's mom briefly and be outside just as the girls from Sydney's cabin were lining up for lunch.

When Sydney caught a glimpse of us, she ran straight for us and jumped into my arms. She was smiling and bubbling over with news. They had played gaga ball; she had mastered the climbing wall and ridden the zipline. She couldn't wait to go tubing. She hadn't slept well, which didn't surprise me, and I noted the dark circles under her eyes. I gave her a squeeze and told her she'd make up for it tonight. Her lower lip trembled slightly as she told us that she'd stood in line the day before at the Ranch House, and her box wasn't there when she got to the counter.

Damn! We had brought the Ranch House snacks in the car with us, thinking they wouldn't be needed until this afternoon. I assured her the box would be waiting for her the next time.

Then it was time for lunch. Sydney gave us both another hug and headed back to join Lizzie and her cabinmates. All in all, she had done great. I watched her small body disappear into the building where they would eat. Again, I said another prayer that all would go well.

It was a short week of camp—from Sunday afternoon to Friday midmorning, but it felt extra long to Joel and me. We enjoyed our getaway in Blowing Rock, and spent peaceful hours walking and talking on the carriage trails at Moses Cone Park. But we missed Sydney. Since we homeschooled, I was used to being with her practically every moment of every day. The hardest part was not being able to talk with her, hear her voice and check in. Parents were allowed to send emails and care packages, which we did, but phone calls were not allowed unless there was an emergency.

Each evening, the camp posted photos from the day, and after our long hikes, Joel and I would scrunch up together on the bed and open my laptop eager to catch a glimpse of our precious girl. Each photo that showed her smiling, laughing, playing with new friends eased our minds. Every day that went by, I felt a little more comfortable, trusting that Sydney was fine, that she was getting enough to eat, that we'd hear if she'd had a gluten exposure.

At the end of the week, since we were already in the mountains, we left Blowing Rock early, so we could pick up Sydney from camp and drive home with her, rather than having her take the bus back to Charlotte.

It was a sweet reunion. We arrived, along with a throng of other parents. Sydney was in her cabin packing. When she saw us at the door, she ran to meet us and give us hugs. She introduced us to several of her cabinmates, and as everyone was getting ready to leave there were lots more hugs all around. I noted Sydney's smile, the slight sunburn on her cheeks, that her hair seemed lighter after several days of being in the sun. She was slim but didn't look emaciated, which was a relief. Her eyes were slightly glazed from tiredness, but she looked happy.

Once in the car, she told us everything—from the bus ride to the moment we arrived back at camp to pick her up. We heard about all the girls in her cabin, her two counselors who were friendly and kind, all the activities—from the Leap of Faith to the zipline to the giant iceberg all the kids climbed on in the lake to the cookouts to the Cookie Mush and on and on.

I listened for places where she might have felt awkward or uncomfortable because of the gluten issues. Did she get enough to eat? How were the meals? Was she able to make s'mores with her gluten-free ingredients? How did it go at the Ranch House?

Yes, she'd gotten enough to eat, though she was hungry at times, especially in the evening when she was used to having a snack before bedtime. She wished she could have had food in her cabin, but they didn't allow that. The meals were mostly what I'd specified but not always. For example, Tuesday's hamburger showed up at dinner instead of lunch. Some of the scrambled eggs I'd packed never appeared, so Sydney filled up on gluten-free cereal. She didn't remember ever seeing the spaghetti I'd made. But she trusted Lizzie's mom, who was always careful to give her chips from our bag or offer her fruit from the salad bar. Sydney didn't actually use all the s'mores ingredients. She just ate the chocolate bar and the marshmallows and forgot about the gluten-free graham crackers. She stood in line with the other campers at the Ranch House and chose whatever she wanted from the box I'd packed.

While the food situation hadn't been perfect, she had managed, even done well. I relaxed, enjoying hearing her tales: she and her partner made it to the top of the climbing wall. Sydney said everyone loved tubing the best. But her cabin only got to go once, due to bad weather. But she and Lizzie rode the tube together and put their thumbs up, signaling the driver of the boat to go as fast as possible. She grinned as she told us this.

A couple of hours later, we pulled into our driveway at home with a tired girl, a duffle bag full of dirty clothes, an empty cooler and the gift of some wonderful camp memories Sydney would always have.

Tenth Birthday

The year was 2011. Sydney was turning ten. Double digits! Birthdays were a favorite and an extra special time of the year. And why not? It was a day to celebrate and be celebrated; there was a party; there were cards and presents to open; family and friends gathered around, dinner was of her choosing and there was cake!

Cake was one of Sydney's all-time favorite treats. She'd gone from vanilla to chocolate and back again, trying to decide her favorite. Birthday cake had a special significance to Sydney, probably because she'd grown up (since her diagnosis at age five) watching other people eat it at parties. There were lavish Cinderella cakes, scrumptious ice cream cakes filled with cookies and cream, double and triple-tiered birthday cakes swirled with colorful, mouth-watering icing, butter cream frosted slices of wedding cake and so much more. All of which she could look at but not eat, while everyone around her feasted.

As a noncook, I couldn't compete. Instead of indulging in her friends' birthday cakes, Sydney unwrapped a gluten-free muffin that I had carefully frosted with safe icing and dashed a handful of gluten-free sprinkles or chocolate chips on top. It was better than nothing. But it wasn't cake.

However, on her tenth birthday, Miss Audrey, a dear friend of the family, had baked a special gluten-free cake and designed it to Sydney's specifications. It was a rectangular-shaped cake with an orange dog face in the middle (depicting our new golden retriever Sunny) and four cat faces—one in each corner—because Sydney had been obsessed with cats since she was a toddler and first buried her nose in the fur of Tatter, my old calico kitty.

The cake had rows of pink and orange decoration icing around the sides. It was not only gluten-free, but it was dairy- and corn-free with a corner that was free of any food dyes, so that Sydney's friend Lauren-Kate could indulge with us. I had offered to make cupcakes that Lauren-Kate could eat. But my daughter wanted her to have part of the real thing—actual birthday cake—what Sydney had been denied so many times herself. Miss Audrey was up to the challenge. It was a glorious cake—one that Sydney *and* all her friends could eat.

First, though, there was pizza, another of Sydney's favorite foods, and one that she'd been forbidden to eat, except for the home-made variety with safe toppings sitting atop the cardboard-like crust I'd found at the local health food store. But for her birthday, Joel had ordered up a special treat: gluten-free pizza from the head chef at his golf club.

In my usual fashion, I probed around to make sure the chef knew what he was doing, and he assured Joel that he did. "They do gluten free all the time, and the pastry chef who has celiac will be making the dough," Joel told me. If anyone understood the dangers of cross contamination, someone who had celiac would. I heaved a sigh of relief that, first off, Sydney could indulge in one of her favorite foods on her birthday, and second, that I didn't have to make it.

When the boxes of pizza arrived, I could see the look of glee on Sydney's face. Just the mere fact that it looked like the kind of pizza that people without allergies ate brought her joy. It had the same pools of oil glistening among the pepperoni and cheese, and the aroma of fresh-baked crust was divine.

Pizza for everyone! The moms and the kids at the party all grabbed slices and the food disappeared quickly. But no one enjoyed the pizza more than Sydney. This was her day, and she wasn't going to miss the opportunity to relish this food. She ate one piece and then another and another, until her tiny stomach had room for only one more thing—cake!

116

The kids gathered around and sang "Happy Birthday" as Sydney smiled. She asked for a corner of cake with one of the cat faces on it and a scoop of ice cream on the side. I served it to her with delight. Because of my own issues with sugar and my concerns about diabetes—the fact that it ran in families, and that people who had celiac had an added risk factor—I didn't offer many sweet desserts at our table. But on this day, I wanted to treat our daughter. What could it hurt?! And again, Sydney relished the sugary moment, licking the icing from around her lips.

Two hours later, after the presents had been opened, the last games had been played, goodbyes had been said and the leftover cake and pizza had been put away, the phone rang. Everyone but Sydney's grandparents had gone home; they were planning to pick up gluten-free "to go" meals from Outback for the family to share for a late dinner.

When I picked up the phone, I heard Miss Audrey's voice: "How's the birthday girl? Did she enjoy the cake?" As I regaled my friend with the story of Sydney's excitement over the cake, I beckoned my daughter to the phone.

Sydney seemed reluctant to talk, and I whispered, "It's Miss Audrey!" She always enjoyed talking with Audrey, so I was surprised when she dragged her feet. "Don't forget to thank her for the cake," I whispered.

Sydney obediently took the phone and slowly walked upstairs. I paused in my kitchen cleaning to listen to her side of the conversation. Sydney's voice was soft. She thanked Audrey and said a few yeses and uh huhs. This was not their normally spirited exchange. I decided that Sydney must be exhausted from the day.

When Sydney padded back downstairs to give me the phone, her face was solemn. "Are you okay, Sweetie?" I asked.

"My tummy doesn't feel good."

"Oh, dear," I said. "I'm sorry. You probably overdid it." Sydney's normal diet was so healthy that it made sense that she would feel a little sick to her stomach after the day's indulgences. Sydney leaned her head against me. "I probably ate too much pizza."

"How many pieces did you have?" I asked, smiling.

She hesitated. "Five."

"Five slices!" No wonder she was feeling bad. "With cake AND ice cream?"

"Yeah."

"That's a lot for one small body," I said, looking into her brown eyes.

"But it was so good, Mommy."

I gave her a hug. "I know, honey. It's okay. Why don't you just rest a little bit, and hopefully you'll feel better."

Sydney picked up a stuffed calico kitten that one of her friends had given her and wandered into her bedroom. A moment later, I heard a gagging sound and then Sydney crying: "Momma, I threw up!"

I rushed over and saw sweat beading on her pale face. She was already gagging again and moving towards the bathroom. I followed her in and watched as she heaved the contents of her stomach into the porcelain bowl. Afterwards, I held her slight body in mine, washed her face with a warm towel as my mind reeled. Maybe Sydney's system couldn't handle all the sugar, all the pizza. Anyone could be nauseous after eating so much. But I sensed this was something more. I remembered the nutritionist sharing stories of her daughter's constant vomiting.

"How are you doing, Sweetie?" I looked into her face and saw misery. We waited. A few moments later she threw up again.

"I don't want to be sick," she cried. "It's my birthday!"

"I know, honey. I'm so sorry." I washed her face again and brought a chair into the bathroom. She sat on my lap and laid her head back against me. Each time she felt her stomach lurch, she stood up and bent over the toilet. Joel and his parents peeked in, then stepped back, their faces etched with worry.

Sydney gagged again and again, every few minutes until her stomach was completely emptied. And she continued dry heaving. It was as if her digestive system was trying to empty itself of any trace of whatever had offended it. It had to be gluten. But how? We'd been so careful.

"It hurts!" she wailed softly.

I gave her small sips of water to wash out her mouth, and she continued throwing up until a yellow liquid came up, which I later learned was bile. I held her and prayed for the vomiting to end, wondering how much more of this her body could take. It continued for two full hours until finally she was so weak, she was almost asleep in my arms. I half-carried her to her bed with a large Tupperware bowl and sat with her as she gradually drifted off.

That night, Joel and I discussed the food. I was sure she'd had a gluten exposure, and not a small one.

We knew the cake had been safe. Miss Audrey had made other cakes for Sydney and was well aware of the dangers of gluten. It had to be the pizza. Was the dough full of wheat? Joel was angry, and he called the head chef who assured him again that the club's pastry chef who had celiac himself had made the dough. It had to be safe. I asked (through Joel) what the ingredients were. The chef named them off one by one. Everything sounded okay. But I knew it was possible to make even a small mistake: leftover flour on the pans, a serving spoon that had been cross-contaminated.

Not everyone knew the subtleties and the dangers of gluten, even those who claimed to understand gluten-free cooking. I asked Joel to investigate further, so the next day he emailed the head chef and asked him about the ingredients in the pizza sauce. Joel read to me from the chef's email, "Tomatoes, olive oil, modified food starch...."

"Stop!" I said, holding up my hand. "That's it. Modified food starch!"

"What?" Joel looked at me with a question in his eyes. "Modified food starch?"

"Yes," I said. "Modified food starch often has wheat in it, unless a label specifically says what the starch is." I groaned. I was angrier with myself than with the chef. I had trusted an unknown source, allowed our family to take this kind of chance, and instead of Sydney's birthday ending with just a pleasantly (and maybe overly) full tummy, it ended with her being horribly and painfully sick.

It was a lesson we would not soon forget.

More Travels

$\mathcal{A}$ s the months passed and we made more trips, I began to get the hang of packing and preparing food. I kept a packing list on my computer and updated it each time we went somewhere new. It not only included basic foods and condiments, but additional items such as our own frying pan and spatula, a thin plastic cutting board, paper plates and plastic silverware so we could easily eat on the road. I even had a list of emergency restaurants or grocery stores and their locations in case we needed to stop and pick up food.

Sydney and I made a couple of trips to the beach with friends. The moms were always supportive and easy to work with. Most of the time, they were willing to eat "the way we did" for a long weekend, or at least the bulk of the meals were gluten-free. I enjoyed cooking with these friends and learned a few domestic tips and new recipes working side-by-side in the kitchen with them.

The kids sometimes made up for their "clean eating" by indulging in candy and wheat-filled snacks between meals. Sydney would have liked to join them, but she knew she couldn't. All in all, though, these trips were a blessing that helped us feel less isolated and segregated by gluten.

A couple of times a year, I took a writing retreat for a few days with my friend Gilda, who was also gluten-free. These trips were the easiest. I could pack one small cooler with a couple of eggs, cooked chicken, broccoli, lettuce, celery and a bag of almonds and be set for two days and two nights. Gilda packed her own cooler with similar ingredients.

The hardest part of the trip was the list I had to write for Joel and Sydney, though I usually just cooked a big meal of spaghetti or made a gluten-free pot pie the night before leaving and put the leftovers in the fridge for them.

During these trips, Gilda and I were more interested in writing than eating, so we kept things simple. We would eat breakfast together and often have a period of silence during the day where we focused heavily on our work. Sometimes we ate lunch or dinner together, heating up our chicken and broccoli but avoiding any hard-core cooking. We took a walk before the sun went down, then we were back at work. As long-time creative friends, we both felt nourished through our conversation and our writing. And it was a joy to be able to retreat with someone who ate the same way I did.

The summer after Sydney's tenth birthday, in addition to the annual trip to Lake George, our family took a side trip to Maine to visit cousins and explore the beautiful landscape. As in the past, I packed a cooler full of meat, vegetables and condiments that were safe for us. Our cousins, who owned a lovely bed and breakfast on the coast and would have been happy to serve us five-star meals, accepted our needs around food with grace and welcomed us and our cooler of gluten-free food.

It was around this same time that we began making our annual trip to Fripp Island with Joel's family. His parents—Sally and Anton—generously rented a large house for the entire Campanella clan, which included us, Joel's two brothers and their families. I planned to bring a couple of coolers for the week and was a little concerned about the co-mingling of food. But my worries turned out to be unnecessary as Sally designated certain shelves of the refrigerator and areas of the kitchen as "gluten free." Having witnessed Sydney's gluten exposure on her tenth birthday, she didn't want it repeated.

Sydney's grandparents were so vigilant about keeping food separate that they asked me to cook all of our own meals. While I was happy to do it, I was also a little sad not to get a break from cooking for at least a few meals. I'll admit I whined a bit, especially when everyone else got to order out for pizza. Of course, it was no one's fault; it was just a part of our new normal—one to which I was still having trouble adjusting.

While we thoroughly enjoyed our long, relaxing days on the beach and the opportunity to spend time with the rest of the family, the hardest part of these trips turned out to be the fact that we ate differently. We were confronted by it at every meal. Sydney looked longingly at her cousins' pizza slices, bowls of ice cream, bags of cookies and chips.

Anton, who was the resident shopper, made every effort to find gluten-free treats for Sydney. But there just wasn't much available at the small, coastal grocery stores. The crackers didn't compare, the cookies had a cardboard texture, the ice cream was plain vanilla (instead of cookies and cream), and on and on.

It wasn't the end of the world. Far from it. We knew we were blessed. Being with family was way more important than what we ate. And we were thrilled to be enjoying time together in a beautiful beach paradise. However, we still couldn't help but be aware that gluten had once again wedged itself between us and everyone else.

Maundy Thursday

I n the spring of 2013, when Sydney was eleven, I took a writing retreat at the beach. The plan was that I would go down on Thursday, and Joel and Sydney would join me after a few days. It was a perfect setup as we had rented my best friend's mother's beach condo. It was oceanfront, beautifully decorated and filled with warm memories. The condo also happened to be located near where I had lived as a teenager, which was an extra bonus.

As a writer, I'd gotten into the habit of taking a few days for myself each year to relax and unwind, nourish my introverted tendencies and work on any writing projects that were important to me. This year, I was doing a final revision for my memoir, *Motherhood: Lost and Found,* a story about my mother's descent into Alzheimer's at the same time I was trying to become a mom and struggling through a series of miscarriages.

My editor had given me a CD of our meeting where we discussed her suggested changes. I had listened to it on the drive to the coast, letting her ideas wash over me and enjoying thoroughly immersing myself in the manuscript again.

Before leaving for the beach, I had followed the usual routine. In addition to packing for myself, I had written an outline of activities for Joel and Sydney to follow. I did this every time I went away, though each year the outline was gradually getting less detailed. It still included a schedule for them to follow and menu suggestions for meals I had cooked and stored in the fridge for them. I smiled as I thought of how Sydney was becoming just as responsible as Joel. She knew exactly what was safe and often reminded her dad of what was on the outline. My detailed notes were no longer necessary.

I had strategically planned my trip around March Madness, so I could escape the basketball mania that overtakes our home during the NCAA tournament. I exhaled with relief knowing that I would enjoy doing my work and being in nature while both Joel and Sydney would have a great time watching basketball together.

The only thing other than basketball on their schedule was a Maundy Thursday dinner, where people were meeting at our church with crockpots of soup for a service that would celebrate the Last Supper. Joel and Sydney would bring the crockpot of soup I had prepared for them and have an easy dinner of soup, salad and gluten-free rolls provided by the church. I had even packed them each a gluten-free brownie to enjoy after dinner.

When I arrived at the condo, the first thing I did was open the blinds so I could take in the view—a beautiful strip of blue green water just beyond the dunes and the maritime forest. I set up my computer on the dining room table where I could pause and look out the window whenever I raised my eyes from my screen.

I got to work right away, not wanting to waste a moment. I would be here by myself for two nights and three days, just enough time to unpack the revisions I was considering and weave important strands into my book.

My editor was encouraging me to explore some deeper emotions in a few of the chapters, and this was the perfect time to do it. My mother had been gone a few years, and here I had the mental space to unravel whatever came up as I probed and journaled my way towards words that would capture the essence of our relationship.

Just before dinner, I took a short break to walk on the beach and called Joel and Sydney. They were in a hurry, rushing out the door to make it to the Maundy Thursday service. "We're doing great!" said Joel. "Don't worry about us!" echoed Sydney. The conversation was brief, but it was nice to hear their voices.

The ocean air was cool and brisk, the salt air wrapped around me reminding me of my high school years on the coast. The condo where I was staying was just steps away from the complex of apartments, one of which my parents rented after we moved here from Panama. I was fifteen at the time, a few years older than my daughter, and I felt raw and vulnerable, having experienced the loss of friends and beloved horses when my father, who was in the military, was transferred away from the Canal Zone.

My mother did her best to comfort me, though it must have been like trying to pet a porcupine. Still, her presence was a balm even if I had a hard time expressing any appreciation for her at the time.

This was one of the reasons I looked forward to staying in this condo. I felt close to my mother here. Memories of her surfaced as I scoured the beach for shells and studied the waves in search of dolphin fins. I wanted to plumb these authentic emotions for my memoir.

When I came back to the condo, I ate a quick dinner and worked as the sky evolved from china blue to peach to sapphire. I moved from the dining room table to a chair in the living room as I changed chapters. Holding my laptop on my crossed legs, tears formed as I thought of how much I needed my mother after Sydney was born. I allowed myself to dive deeply into the complicated emotions I felt at that time. I grieved over her disease. Our roles had reversed, and I had become her caretaker. Yet, I was grateful for her presence, the warmth of her smile, the love that lit up her face even when she couldn't say my name. I added new scenes, struggling to capture these feelings.

The hours ticked away, and when I looked up at the clock, it was late, almost midnight. I closed my laptop, satisfied with the day's work and excited about what I planned to tackle in the morning.

In the bedroom, I laid my head on the pillow and thought of Joel and Sydney. They were no doubt staying up late watching basketball. Sydney normally went to bed much earlier, but since she was homeschooled, she could always sleep in. Besides, this was special Daddy/daughter time.

As I closed my eyes, I heard a sound. It gradually got louder, and I sat up. My phone. I wasn't worried. It was probably Joel calling to say goodnight since we hadn't had much time to talk earlier.

When I answered I was surprised to hear my sweet girl's voice. "Mommy, I'm sick."

Adrenaline pierced my body, but I kept my voice calm. "Oh, Sweetie. What's going on?"

"I've been throwing up." And I heard her tears begin to flow.

"Oh, honey, I'm so sorry." This was my worst nightmare—not being home when Sydney needed me.

"Daddy didn't want me to call you. He said you were busy writing," and she gave a quiet sob.

"You know you can call me any time."

"I knew you'd say that." I heard her sniffling.

"Where's Dad?" I asked.

"He's watching the game."

"Sweetie, I'm so sorry I'm not there to take care of you. Tell me what happened."

Sydney proceeded to tell me how she and Joel had gone to the Maundy Thursday service. They had eaten the soup I had prepared, and each of them had some bread that had been passed around in baskets labeled gluten free. After the baskets had been cleared from the tables, Sydney had gone back for one more piece of bread. She saw the gluten-free label in the basket, but she knew as soon as she took a bite, that the labels must have been mixed up when the tables were cleared.

"The texture of bread just felt different in my mouth," she said. "On the way home," she continued. "I had a bad taste in the back of my mouth, and I started to feel anxious. We got home and turned on the basketball. We watched the end of the Florida Gulf Coast Game, and I felt nauseous. I was hoping I was just really hungry. After the game was over, I went to the kitchen to try to eat a pretzel. I bit into it and couldn't even swallow it." She had to run to the bathroom.

She called out to Joel to tell him she'd thrown up. "Dad said he'd come check on me after the first media timeout." My husband is a wonderful husband and father, but he's not the person you want around when you're sick.

"My poor sweetheart," I moaned softly. "What did you do?"

"I kept throwing up, over and over. Dad said to stay in the bathroom, so I wouldn't make a mess, and he went back to watch more basketball.

I was scared to leave. When I finally felt like I might not get sick again, I snuck over and grabbed the phone."

"I'm so glad you called me." I sighed.

"Mommy, I need you." The pleading in Sydney's voice cut straight through my heart. If I could have poured myself through the phone I would have. I thought about getting in the car right that minute and driving through the early morning hours. But I was six hours away. By the time I got home, the crisis would be past, and she would be asleep. My arms ached to hold her, every fiber in my being wanted to enfold, comfort and protect her.

"Oh, honey, I know. I'm here. You can call me any time, day or night. I'm sending you the biggest hug possible through the phone."

It was early Friday morning. I would see Sydney on Saturday afternoon, in a day and a half. But when you feel sick, you need your mother now, not in two days. How I wished I could teleport myself back to my daughter's side to comfort and watch over her, to keep her from harm.

I stayed on the phone as long as Sydney wanted to talk. She didn't feel good, and she was scared she might start getting sick again. She alternated between crying softly and telling me how bad she felt. I suggested she try eating some ice chips to keep from getting dehydrated.

At one point, she gave the phone to Joel, and I couldn't hide my exasperation: "You sent her to the bathroom and went back to watch the game?! And you told her she couldn't call me!" I accused. He murmured that he knew I needed time to work. Even in the heat of the moment, I couldn't stay mad at him. Joel was not a natural nurturer, though he loved his family passionately. He just showed it in different ways. He was the coach of Sydney's basketball team; he had urged me to go on this retreat because he knew how important writing was to me, and he had cleared his schedule (for the most part) and truly enjoyed spending one-on-one time with his daughter.

"Joel, if this ever happens again, please just go into the bathroom *with* Sydney." I vehemently instructed. "At least check on her!"

I spent the next day working on my manuscript nonstop, except for my periodic calls home. I talked with Joel in the morning before Sydney woke up and learned that she went back and finished watching the game with him. Joel said her eyes were half-closed and she leaned against him the whole time. It was a tender image, although part of me wished he could have turned off the TV and encouraged her to go to bed. Isn't that what good parents are supposed to do? Especially when your child has spent two hours hugging the porcelain bowl. But another part of me gave thanks for this diversion of basketball, a sport they both loved. I hoped somehow it would help to soothe the wound my absence had created.

In some ways, it seemed uncanny that I was spending the day deepening the emotional resonance of a memoir about my own mother. One of the layers I was working on was making sure the book showed how much I missed my mother after Sydney was born. She was present in body, but with Alzheimer's taking over her mind, she wasn't able to enter into the challenges of caring for an infant with me. I couldn't ask her questions; I couldn't receive the comfort of her stories. If she couldn't remember what was happening in my life, she couldn't ride the emotional currents with me. I felt alone during those years.

The fact that Sydney was alone when she needed me sent a dagger of pain into my chest. Part of me knew this situation was different. I was there for Sydney most of the time, just not physically present for a few days. I would see her soon. She would get over this, be fine, maybe not even remember the details of last night's ordeal. But another part of me understood more clearly than ever the danger that gluten posed to my child. I would never have the power to plan or foresee every situation, to protect her from harm.

Around midday, I called home to talk with Sydney. Her voice sounded a little smaller than usual. She had eaten eggs for breakfast, but her stomach was sore from all the throwing up. I suggested some soothing foods to try, and I told her I couldn't wait to see her on Saturday. I knew she was still missing me, but she perked up when I asked about her basketball bracket. Joel was upbeat as usual, reminding me that the games were starting again.

I worked deep into the night and early the next morning finishing up my revisions for the most part. Actually, I just had to tell myself to stop because I could easily overwork a manuscript if I wasn't careful. I made the decision to put it aside, so that I still had time to do some journaling and take a walk on the beach. I wanted to be refreshed and ready to welcome my family with open arms and a full heart. I counted the minutes until I would see them again.

When I heard Joel's car pull up that afternoon, I ran down the stairs to meet them. Sydney's door opened in a flash and she was in my arms! I couldn't help but take in her physical condition. Her face looked almost bruised, and her eyes were sunken. They had a glassy look (too much TV) and the dark circles under them told me she hadn't had enough sleep. I hugged her small body to mine and felt her ribs.

I silently cursed this thing called celiac that had made my daughter vulnerable and the gluten that attacked her when I was away.

Dr. G

*A*s Sydney and I found our stride in the homeschooling world, and I was no longer a caregiver for my mother, I had time to turn my attention to my own health. I was approaching menopause. Each time, I had my annual physical, my doctor told me I had borderline hypothyroidism, which meant my thyroid was sluggish. I would usually have my TSH level checked and then rechecked six months later. The levels improved enough that my doctor didn't recommend anything further. Yet, I still didn't feel great.

It wasn't the bloating, tiredness or brain fog that came along with eating wheat. I'd had years of serious sleep deprivation when I was caring for my mother and Sydney at the same time, and I still wasn't sleeping well, due to fluctuating hormones. More often than not, I woke in the morning and felt as if I lived through the day with a scrim of pain—in my head and behind my eyes. I didn't realize my adrenals were shot and that there was a complex connection between my adrenal and thyroid glands. Autoimmune disorders such as Hashimoto's, which is a form of hypothyroidism, occur when your immune system produces antibodies that attack your own tissues.

I learned about all of this when I went to see Dr. G, a local functional medicine practitioner who had a reputation for working outside the box. I had called around interviewing a handful of medical and alternative doctors about their approach to hypothyroidism and chose Dr. G because I liked that he treated patients with natural supplements.

Joel and I had been going to an acupuncturist who we loved for years, and although I liked my traditional doctor, I didn't have a lot of faith in the American medical system, which focused more on disease symptoms rather than an awareness of the whole person. My body was sensitive, and it always responded better to natural treatments than medicine or pharmaceuticals.

Dr. G's tests revealed that I had Hashimoto's. One of the first things he wanted to do was remove any allergens from my diet. "I'm already gluten free," I pronounced proudly. He went on to say that most people who thought they were gluten free weren't really because of all the hidden sources of gluten in foods. "Oh, I've got this one," I maintained. "Our daughter has celiac."

Okay. Check. Gluten was not a problem then. But did I know that other foods such as dairy could cause an inflammatory response similar to gluten in the body? Umm...I knew a little bit about that. Our acupuncturist had long ago educated Joel and me about the dangers of consuming too much dairy. Yet, Dr. G went further, saying that even the tiniest amount of dairy (like gluten) could set off a reaction in the body that could last for as long as six months. Six months!

One of the first things he did was give me a blood test that would show to which of the common allergens my body was reacting. Gluten and dairy showed up, which was no surprise. Then he put me on a strict diet where I avoided all allergens. He also discovered that I had been living with a parasite in my digestive tract. After six or eight weeks of clean eating and adding certain parasite-ridding supplements to my diet, I began to feel as if I was awakening from a long sleep.

Joel, who was always eager to find new ways to improve his golf game, joined me in working with Dr. G. Cutting out gluten had helped him feel better, so why not take the next step? He was thrilled to find that when he cut out dairy completely his regular flareups of arthritis seemed to vanish and that his golf swing was as smooth and supple as ever.

During the next year, Joel and I discussed the possibility of bringing Sydney to Dr. G. She was definitely tired of doctor visits, and I didn't want to do anything unnecessary. But both Joel and I had discovered new allergies and how the removal of them were improving our quality of life. If dairy was an inflammatory for both of us, and she was our child, wasn't it likely that she might have the same allergy?

I hated to introduce even the thought of one more allergen. Wasn't gluten enough? It had already separated Sydney in so many ways from many of her friends. But what if dairy was negatively affecting her health, causing a drag on her organs, keeping her from feeling her best? Just like with gluten, she might not know it until it was gone from her regular diet. As her parents, we felt we owed it to our daughter to at least check this out.

Sydney reluctantly submitted to one more blood test. She had seen me going in for weekly appointments as I worked on improving my hypothyroidism, and I assured her that she wouldn't have to visit over and over with Dr. G. We'd simply get the results from him and figure out where to go from there.

It was no surprise to discover that Sydney's test showed she was allergic to dairy. For Joel and me, adapting to a dairy-free lifestyle hadn't been hard, especially compared to eliminating gluten. We could drink almond or coconut milk instead of cow's milk. We were already shopping in health food stores. Like gluten, dairy lurked in processed foods, so we just had to scan the labels for one more allergen. Instead of milk chocolate, there was dark chocolate or bars made with rice milk. It seemed that dairy allergies were more prevalent than gluten ones, so foods—for the most part—were clearly labeled.

One problem would be pizza. Sydney was used to eating homemade pizza with rice cheese. But the rice cheese contained casein, a protein found in dairy and something that was a definite "no-no" according to Dr. G.

She didn't mind having almond milk with her cereal. And I was already substituting almond or coconut milk in most recipes. The worst thing would be giving up her favorite ice cream—Breyer's Vanilla—which was gluten free, but full of dairy.

We went on a long search trying to find replacements that would feel like a treat. Joel was content with ice cream made with coconut milk, but Sydney didn't care for the flavor of coconut. We tried various frozen desserts made from rice and almond milk. We even purchased a homemade ice cream maker, and I (the noncook) attempted several nondairy ice cream recipes. Those concoctions turned out to be strange-tasting, soupy combinations of fruit and icy milk. Perhaps someone more skilled than I would have had better luck. But I struck out at discovering a substitute that matched the delicious creaminess of Breyer's. Not even close.

Eventually, we found a brand of frozen dessert—chocolate Almond Dream—that Sydney grew to enjoy, as long as no one else was eating dairy ice cream within her vicinity.

Last Year of Camp

S ydney went back to the same camp she had gone to for two more summers. The second time she had a good experience, similar to the first. But the third year, when we expected it to be "old hat," things fell apart.

It shouldn't have been a surprise that the issue turned out to be food. During this visit to camp, Sydney had to adjust to being not only gluten free, but dairy free as well. I didn't think it would make much difference because (as in the past) I would be supplying all of her food. But, the doctor had warned Sydney to stay away from anything containing milk, and unbeknownst to us, Sydney feared that if she accidentally had a tiny bit of dairy, she'd have the same awful reaction that she had to gluten. This wasn't the case. Dairy would cause inflammation in her system, showing up mostly as congestion and minor digestive issues. But it would not trigger the cycle of throwing up. Sydney didn't know this, which left her more anxious than in previous years.

Timing also turned out to be a huge factor. Sydney's third year of camp was scheduled at the beginning of the summer, instead of at the end (like the first two camps she had attended). I didn't take notice of this or have any inkling that it would be an issue. Everything ran smoothly in the dining hall by the end of summer. But, apparently, the first week of camp was when the kinks were ironed out. Imagine the head cook instructing a handful of teenagers and a few moms about how to feed three-hundred kids three meals a day for the first time.

So even though I had packed our cooler in the same way I'd done in the past, the kitchen staff was still learning the ropes. And having a camper with celiac had not registered high on their radar (perhaps because I hadn't made as big a deal about it as before). Also, Penny, Sydney's friend's mother, wasn't working in the kitchen during this session of camp.

But none of these things set off warning bells in my mind. They only began to ring later, after I learned that several of her meals were mixed up. Sydney knew there was a problem, but as a quiet, unassuming eleven-year-old, she wasn't able to convince the staff that they'd made a mistake. And, wisely, she didn't trust that the food they brought to her was safe.

By the end of the week, Sydney was so nervous (and hungry) that she couldn't sleep. She asked her counselor if she could call us. Joel and I were in Blowing Rock again when Joel's cell phone rang. It was the camp director. Joel talked with him first and then handed the phone to me. He told us that our daughter was very upset and wanted to go home. His voice was pleasant, but firm. He advised me not to talk with Sydney directly, that it would make things worse, and he urged us not to let her go home early. I listened and understood that he had a lot of experience dealing with homesick kids at camp. He clearly meant well. But I'd never received a call from anyone telling me Sydney was upset and crying. This was not like her. She enjoyed camp, and even if she *was* homesick, she wouldn't call us unless there was a major problem. Sydney wasn't one to bring attention to herself...ever. Unless she felt unsafe.

I needed to hear what was going on from Sydney. So, I told the camp director I wanted to talk with my daughter.

Sydney was in tears on the phone. "You've got to come get me," she wailed. "Please."

"What's going on, Sweetie?" I asked. And Sydney blurted out that the staff told her that I hadn't packed food for some of her meals. They brought her plates of pasta, meat and vegetables she didn't recognize, so she didn't know if they were gluten and dairy free or not.

"Oh, honey. I'm so sorry. You know I packed food for every meal. And even some extras."

"I know you did. But they said you didn't!" Sydney said between sobs.

"Let me talk with the director again. Maybe I can explain."

"I've tried to," she said. "They don't understand. No one understands. Mommy, I'm so scared that I'll get sick again like I did on Maundy Thursday, and you won't be here!"

Sydney's words cut straight through my heart, and I felt her fear. What child wouldn't be scared? She knew what gluten could do to her, and she was wise enough—even at the tender age of eleven—to know most people were cavalier about the dangers of wheat because they hadn't gone through what she had.

When the director came back on the phone, I took a deep breath and told him Sydney's concern about getting sick, how the smallest crumb of wheat could make her seriously ill for hours and that the staff had mixed up her meals. I tried to sound calm and knowledgeable, so he wouldn't think I was a hysterical mother. The director was kind, but immovable. He didn't get it. He thought everything would be fine, that she should stay at camp. Even as I was trying to help him understand, I knew he never would, unless he had experienced the symptoms of celiac disease himself. This kind of anxiety around food didn't arise for no reason. It was only a few months ago that Sydney had thrown up over and over for two hours straight, after eating a small piece of bread. She threw up so much that her entire digestive tract was inflamed, and yellow bile was coming out of her. She didn't want a repeat. For good reason. Especially without Mom.

I asked to talk to Sydney again. She continued to cry on the phone. "You've got to come get me tonight. I can't stay here any longer." I held the phone out, so Joel could hear her. We looked at each other, stricken by the fear in her voice.

As I spoke soothingly to Sydney, she began to calm down. She continued to beg me to come get her. My mind circled the options. Tomorrow was the last full day of camp. It would be miserable for Sydney if she was hungry and anxious the whole day. I wanted her to know she could count on us to protect her. I also wanted her to know she was strong enough to survive a difficult situation. It really didn't feel safe for her to stay at camp. Unlike previous years, the kitchen staff was mostly teenagers, and I couldn't expect them to understand the severity of an exposure. Just like I couldn't expect the director to understand Sydney's anxiety.

But it was late. I quickly weighed the pros and cons of rescuing Sydney. I didn't want to create a bigger issue by rushing to her side. But I knew my daughter. She wasn't a whiner or someone who cried wolf. I asked her if she could make it through the night. She sniffled and said she could. I swallowed and told her we'd be there in the morning. As I hung up the phone, I knew it was the right decision.

After getting home, Joel, Sydney and I discussed the issues at camp. That's when we realized the problems inherent with a camp week scheduled at the beginning of the summer. It didn't really matter. The damage was done. Camp had lost its appeal to Sydney. Part of me was sad that it had ended this way; another part of me simply accepted that this was life. It didn't always turn out the way we hoped. Besides, Sydney was growing and changing. Three years of camp were enough for now. Maybe someday she'd go again. Or maybe not. Either way, she'd be fine. And I was thankful Sydney hadn't become ill at camp. It might have taught the staff a lesson. But it would have been awful for our girl.

One of the lessons I learned that week was how much I trusted my daughter. I'd always known she was well-grounded and smart, a hard-working and conscientious child. But I gained a new and better understanding of how well she intuitively knew herself. It was a strength I admired and was a little in awe of because it seemed to come so naturally.

The anxiety from camp lingered through the summer. Sydney had stomachaches that made her uncomfortable and sometimes brought her to tears. I hoped that just being home in her normal environment would heal whatever was ailing her. But the stomachaches persisted. Sometimes they were so bad, Sydney would hold her tummy and moan. I took her to a pediatric gastroenterologist, and after drawing multiple vials of blood, she diagnosed Sydney with intestinal spasms.

"Spasms can be quite painful," the doctor said.

She wrote a prescription and handed it to me. "This should take care of it."

After three or four doses of medication over the next couple of weeks, the pain faded as mysteriously as it had appeared. Yet, Sydney's experience at camp would stay with us all for much longer. Having celiac in a world where people ate wheat would remain a challenge. However, I trusted that her gift of self-knowledge would help her on the journey.

Final Years of Homeschooling

We homeschooled Sydney for six years, from second grade through seventh. While homeschooling was demanding at times, I would never give up the experience. I felt blessed to share that time with my daughter, to learn more about who she was, to make memories and guide her. If she hadn't had celiac disease, we might have never gone down the homeschooling path. Going gluten free had actually drawn our family together.

Joel had always played an important role in Sydney's life. But homeschooling allowed him to spend even more time with her. We'd always made family time a priority. We spent afternoons at the park and played games together most evenings.

Most days, after Sydney's schoolwork was done, she'd play basketball with her dad. Sometimes, I'd take a walk, enjoying a half hour to myself. Other times, they'd ask me to referee one of their games. During March Madness, they watched basketball endlessly. When the Final Four was on, I'd make gluten-free dinners we could eat together in front of the TV.

On cold, rainy days or during hot summer afternoons and evenings, we'd gather around our living room table and play board games as Sydney snacked on popcorn, apples or tortilla chips. Joel and I were both quite competitive, and it wasn't long before Sydney caught on. She could figure out any game that had a strategy and beat us soundly in *Parcheesi, Monopoly* or *10 Days in Europe.* As a writer, I usually won the word games, while Joel, who understood calculus and became Sydney's math tutor, remained the champion in games that required math skills such as Yahtzee.

As homeschool parents, it was easy to introduce Sydney to our passions—basketball and golf for Joel, and horseback riding and writing for me. In addition to playing basketball and watching games together, Joel coached Sydney's Upwards basketball team for three years during fourth, fifth and sixth grades. The team met for practice once a week and played games every Saturday. Afterwards, I (or one of the other moms) provided snacks for the kids. As the coach's wife, I emailed the other moms and encouraged them to bring fruit and gluten-free food and drinks.

Joel also lured Sydney to the golf course with the promise of a Gatorade (Shhh...don't tell Mom!) and the opportunity to beat him soundly by creating a handicap system that favored her. For a couple of years, they played nine holes off and on, once every other month or so, which thrilled my husband.

Sydney shared my love of animals. It didn't matter the size; if it had fur, Sydney was attracted to it. As a toddler, I'd find her draped over my calico cat, who was napping in her basket. I have photos of Sydney at the age of four happily sitting on a pony named Cinnamon. A friend who was leasing our barn owned the elderly pony, and Sydney considered Cinnamon "hers." After Cinnamon passed away, we filled Sydney's life with other animals. For her seventh birthday, we went to the pet store and picked out a rescue kitten—another calico—named Melia. A few years later, after much begging, we broke down and got Sunny, a golden retriever puppy. Sydney started feeding and adopted a stray cat she called Cinder that showed up at our house. At Christmas, our fireplace was lined with half a dozen stockings—one for each of us and every pet. Our animals were part of the family. So, it wasn't a surprise when Sydney started asking for a pony.

Even though we had our own farm and I had been a riding instructor for much of my life, I didn't want to rush into buying a horse. Sydney was still young, and I knew how much time and commitment horses required. After Sydney and her friend Lauren-Kate turned ten, Karen and I had signed them up for riding lessons at a nearby farm. Of course, my daughter loved them, and her weekly lessons brought back the special bonds I'd had with the horses of my past. I wondered how long it would be before a horse became our next family member.

2 Bars 7 Ranch: A Gluten-Free Vacation

*I*n early August, two months after Sydney's summer camp, we took our first ever gluten-free vacation on a ranch on the border of Colorado and Wyoming. At eleven years old, Sydney was the perfect age to enjoy a week with horses, although I hadn't originally planned for this. Back in the winter, I had just been scouring the internet for a celiac-safe getaway, not even knowing if such a thing existed.

January was a great time to daydream about summer vacations. It was too cold to spend much time outside, and websites with beach scenes and pools were an enticing lure.

Homeschooling had drawn us into a tight family unit, and I wanted us to have a unique experience—something beyond our usual activities and vacations with extended family, an adventure we could share, a trip that would be memorable and fun. I had imagined a destination where I wouldn't have to cook and all our meals would be safe.

I looked up beach and island resorts, studied menus, read reviews written by people with allergies or celiac disease. Sadly, most of them were having a lovely vacation until one of their meals had been contaminated by gluten. Spending a small fortune for a resort vacation where the meals might make Sydney sick was not in my plan.

A few reviews said if you took the time to visit the kitchen and get to know the chef, the chances of "safe dining" were much higher. Being an introvert, it all sounded rather exhausting.

Up until now, I had insisted that if we ever went somewhere, we pack our own food and stay in a place that at a minimum had a kitchenette, so I could control the contents of all the meals. It had worked. Sydney had rarely gotten sick. But I was in desperate need of a break. At least I wanted to dream of taking a break from cooking. And January had been a great month to dream.

I remembered spending a few weeks on a ranch out West with my best friend after we had graduated from college. Lyn and I had worked as wranglers, guiding guests on trail rides through the Rockies on our sturdy Mustangs. The landscape was stark and beautiful, and being surrounded by nature and horses fed my soul.

Just for fun, I plugged into my computer's search engine: ranch, wrangler and Wyoming. Maybe I was hoping to find the website of the ranch where Lyn and I had worked, so I could peruse the scenery and continue my daydream. I didn't. But scanning photos of random horses and ranch life brought a smile to my face.

On a whim I added "gluten free" to my search. To my surprise, 2 Bars 7 Ranch popped up, a ranch that provided a completely gluten-free menu to guests with celiac disease. Could it be? A ranch on the border of Wyoming that offered weekly stays where we could ride every day and be served food that wouldn't make any of us sick? It sounded too good to be true. Not only could we eat safely, but Sydney could spend a week with horses. I would enjoy the riding too, and a week would give me time to assess Sydney's passion and decide if I should look for a horse for her.

I quickly emailed Polly, the owner, and asked a few questions about the food. She wrote back immediately explaining that she had celiac disease. During the summers, she brought in a cook who also had celiac to provide allergy-safe meals for her and some of her guests. They were used to making gluten-free and dairy-free meals. That would not be a problem. If we had any questions, Polly was happy to give me a call.

This wasn't a place that had a menu where we might find one thing that was safe for us to eat. This ranch experience was designed for people like us! I couldn't believe it!

I dialed the number to the ranch to find out if there were any spaces available in late July. Polly said, "No," and my heart sank. Apparently,

2 Bars 7 was popular and filled up with repeat guests. (I could see why!) Most people, Polly said, booked a year or more in advance. My dream of spending a week on a ranch was blowing away like tumbleweed.

"Wait a minute," she murmured into the phone. "There might have been a cancellation…." Polly put me on hold while she looked at her calendar. "Yes, we have one room available in early August. We could put two double beds in there."

I grabbed it!

The deposit check was due right away. Joel, the paramount golfer in the family, wasn't so sure about spending a week on a ranch.

"But you play golf fifty-two weeks of the year," I said to him.

"I know, and I like it that way," he said. "I'll only be able to play fifty-one weeks if we go to Wyoming."

I couldn't tell if he was joking or not. But Joel was used to getting his way. I had to exert a little muscle.

"Listen, I'm not a cook, and I've been cooking three hundred and sixty-five days of the year. I think I deserve a week off."

"Of course, you can take a week off. We could go to a nice golf resort. I'm sure they have something gluten free there."

Joel clearly had not researched the reviews like I had. "I don't want to take a chance with Sydney getting sick. This is her vacation too."

"Besides, Sydney and I love horses. This is a chance for us to do something together as a family. If you don't want to ride, I'm sure there's something else you could do at the ranch." It was time for me to bring the big guns in. "I hear they make some pretty good gluten-free desserts."

"They do?" Joel was now listening.

"Yup." I nodded. "Every night." A week of gluten-free meals prepared by an actual cook *and* gluten-free desserts! I knew my husband and his appetites. This was enough to win him over.

Our time at the ranch turned out to be an amazing experience. Between not having to cook a single meal for a week and being surrounded by horses and miles of undeveloped land, I was in heaven.

Without my having to say a word, Cassandra, the cook, knew we were the gluten-free, dairy-free family. She took us on a tour of the kitchen, showing us the allergen-free areas of the grill, counter and refrigerator. She pointed out where the "safe" bread and snacks were stored. Sometimes she would serve gluten-free, dairy-free meals to everyone, and when she didn't, there would always be a version that was just as tasty made especially for us. And, as I promised Joel, there were desserts. Not the leftover, stale variety that had been stored for months for the handful of guests who were gluten free. But a homemade, delicious one, piping hot from the oven that would magically appear in front of us every night after dinner.

Before each meal, someone rang the dinner bell, which was mounted on a post outside the dining area. Guests would step out of the row of rustic rooms and walk across the dirt road where the horses were led out to pasture each evening. About a dozen people and the wrangler—a cowboy named J.D.—joined us for meals around a large table. Polly introduced us to her daughter Peg saying, "She's a genuine cowgirl."

During our first dinner, J.D. asked about our previous riding experience, and he made us write down our weight so that he could match us up with appropriate horses. Sydney was given Rascal, a cute, medium-sized paint who was a favorite with kids. Because I had taught riding for much of my life, J.D. gave me Vapor, a horse that was used to a more experienced rider. Joel had taken horseback riding lessons early in our marriage in exchange for me playing golf with him, but he didn't want to overextend himself. So, he asked for a "Cadillac" of trail horses. He was given Polito, a horse with a velvety smooth canter who liked to buddy up with my horse.

On our second day, we learned we'd be helping out with an authentic cattle drive. A couple of the guests with no horse experience stayed behind. Knowing we'd be spending several hours in the saddle, we made sure to fill up on breakfast.

We were not disappointed. There was bacon, eggs, gluten-free biscuits and pancakes. Even pastries that were gluten free. Joel made sure to sample everything and had multiple helpings. I began to worry that he should have added ten pounds to the weight he had given to J.D. Hopefully, he wouldn't be too heavy for Polito by the end of the week.

As we mounted our horses, I took in the panorama of scenery—open land extending in every direction, paths through sagebrush, mountain trails and a huge canvas of blue sky etched by clouds. J.D. warned us that we might see wild animals—moose, coyotes, bears and even mountain lions.

J.D. explained how we were to corral the cattle on horseback and guide them from one pasture to another, funneling them through a small gate. When we came upon the herd, J.D. split us up. Joel and I were on the near side with J.D., while Sydney and the others formed a line on the far side. I was a little nervous being separated from Sydney and kept glancing back to check on her. But the other riders kept an eye out for her, and, truth be told, she was probably more comfortable than most of the adults.

Fortunately for our inexperienced group, the cows knew what to do, for the most part. As long as we kept them bottled between our two lines of horses, they placidly made their way to the new pasture, mooing as they ambled along.

But at the bottom of the hill near the gate, J.D. had warned us of a bog. Some of the herd darted into it, lured by the fresh, green grass. J.D. galloped toward Joel and me, yelling, "Get them!"

Joel and Polito moved out of the way as I guided Vapor into the ankle-deep mud and whooped and hollered along with J.D. Vapor showed off his cutting skills, and after a few minutes of excitement, we managed to bring the wandering cows back to the herd. Joel lounged in his Western saddle, capturing the action on his phone until J.D. barked orders: "Catch that one on the right, Joel!" My husband's video was cut short as he shoved his phone in his pocket and got to work.

Once the cows were safely in their new pasture, Joel and I joined up with Sydney. I pulled out a banana and a couple of gluten-free granola bars from my saddle bag to share with my husband and daughter. It had been a fun, active morning, and we were already looking forward to getting back to the ranch for our gluten-free lunch.

We spent every day on horseback enjoying the wilderness. To my surprise, Joel—the golf fanatic—enjoyed his time riding as much as Sydney and I did, even if he did spend much of his time on horseback envisioning golf holes laid out among the rocks and sagebrush.

I particularly appreciated not only knowing that our food was safe, but not having to think about it. Even for a moment. Breakfast, lunch and dinner were delicious, gluten- and dairy-free meals and different every day. Everything from waffles to chicken casseroles and beef stroganoff. Our meals were so filling, there wasn't a great need for snacks, but if we wanted one, we could wander into the kitchen and find fruit or leftover baked goods from the night before.

On one of the last days, we took an all-day trail ride, and without us saying a word, Cassandra rolled up in the chuckwagon (an old station wagon) with a bounty of food that we could eat—sandwiches made with gluten-free bread, packs of gluten-free chips and crackers, even huge chocolate chip cookies that were safe. It was a little slice of heaven.

Joel, Sydney and I felt authentic grief when it was time to leave. Even though we had a couple more days of vacation left to explore the Rockies by car, we couldn't get excited about it. Figuring out what we would eat became a challenge again. The ranch had been a world unto itself. As we shared meals and days on horseback, the other guests, J.D., Polly and Peg had become like family. And we had a special place in our hearts for Cassandra, who had made it possible for us to eat for a week like the rest of the world with no stress or worry.

Sydney had fallen head over heels in love with Rascal. If it was possible, she would have packed him in her suitcase and brought him home. Seeing the deep bond that had developed between the two of them made me know that it wouldn't be long before it was time to begin the search for a horse of her own.

Horses and Going Back to School

*D*uring Sydney's seventh grade year, we discussed the possibility of her playing basketball with a small private school that allowed homeschoolers on their team. We figured it would be a good opportunity for her to improve her basketball skills, meet new people and expand her world. Sydney joined the team and quickly became friends with the other girls. When the season was over, after getting a taste of the social life at a traditional school, Sydney made the decision to apply as a full-time student.

I was both excited for her to have this new opportunity and wary about the gluten minefields that lay ahead. But at thirteen, Sydney was older and had plenty of wisdom about food. Still, I imagined it would be hard to make the transition from the bubble of homeschool—where staying away from gluten had become, for the most part, a nonissue—to classrooms and lunches full of "normal food." In the long term, I knew Sydney would have to face the real world and all its gluten issues sometime, and this sweet school seemed like a good place to start.

After basketball season, while we were still homeschooling, I brought up the idea of finding a horse for Sydney. I'd been mulling the possibility for some time. From my own experience of growing up with horses, I knew that taking care of them encouraged responsibility and a sense of independence along with a deep bond of understanding and compassion. I wanted Sydney to have these gifts.

While we lived on a farm and had a barn, pastures and fencing, taking the step to add horses was a more complicated endeavor than it seemed on the surface. For one thing, it would be a challenge to find the *right* horse—one that was safe for a beginner rider and easy to work around on the ground. I knew every horse had its own unique personality, and many of them had hidden vices. Also, horses were herd animals, which meant you couldn't have just one. And the more horses you had, the more manual labor it took to care for them. Horses required hay and grain twice a day, access to fresh water and safe pastures. If they were stalled part of the day, which ours would be, stalls had to be cleaned daily. Having horses necessitated scheduling around them every day. But chores would teach responsibility, while learning to work with and around horses would encourage self-reliance and provide a sense of accomplishment.

If we were going to have horses, it felt like it was now or never. I didn't want this window in Sydney's life to close before I'd shared my love for these exquisite animals with her. Sydney was excited and at an age where I could count on her to help. Her friend Lauren-Kate was equally passionate about horses, and her mother and I had many conversations during our homeschooling breaks about the details involved to make this dream come true for our girls. I had the barn, the property and the horse experience, while Karen provided enthusiasm, support and additional labor. The four of us spent our afternoons preparing the barn. Karen and I donned masks and cleared cobwebs, mildew and dust from the tack and feed rooms, while the girls emptied the stalls of old hay and brought in wheelbarrow loads of fresh shavings. One warmish late winter day, they sat in the sun and cleaned all my old tack.

I knew how easy it was to fall in love with a horse, whether it was the right one or not. So, I waited until March to begin scanning local Facebook sites for possible horses. Fortunately, I'd done my share of horse training, so I figured even if I couldn't find the perfect beginner pony, I could work with one that was hopefully close to perfect and address any minor behavioral issues.

We also needed a companion horse or pony. I was lucky to come across a Shetland pony named Smokey whose owner was willing to have me "borrow" him for as long as I liked. He was too small to be ridden by anyone other than toddler-sized kids, but he would be a good companion. Lauren-Kate was content to wait before purchasing a horse and would take lessons on the one I found for Sydney.

Foxie, a pale palomino mare, caught my attention the first time I scanned the horse photos on Facebook. She had the same kind look in her dark eyes that I had seen in my old pony Cochise's eyes. Sydney knew her own propensity to fall in love, so she asked me to go visit Foxie the first time without her. I did, and Foxie, who had been a therapy horse for disabled kids, passed my test. She was as calm and gentle as any horse I'd ever seen on the ground. When I rode her, she was obedient and willing—not a plug by any means—and her gaits were smooth and relaxed.

That same week, I brought Sydney, Lauren-Kate and Karen out to see Foxie. The girls brushed her, and Foxie stood without moving a muscle. I helped Sydney tack her up and attached a lunge line to her bridle. This allowed me to keep control of Foxie while Sydney rode her at a walk and a slow trot in a circle around me. Back in the car, as the girls were snacking on apple slices, I asked my daughter what she thought of Foxie. "I love her," she said in a quiet voice.

That was the beginning of a new relationship. Sydney and Foxie were both thirteen. It was the perfect age to fall in love with a horse, and Sydney fell hard. She spent hours grooming Foxie and braiding her mane, while Lauren-Kate did the same with Smokey. I gave riding lessons a few times a week to both girls, keeping Foxie on the lunge line. The mare behaved herself, as if she understood her role was to introduce the girls to the joy of riding. After a month, Lauren-Kate found a horse named Misty to lease, and we brought her to the barn. So, each girl had her own horse to ride.

As spring evolved into summer, we spent our mornings and evenings feeding, cleaning stalls and scrubbing water buckets. I gave lessons to the girls in the cool of the morning or after dinner when the sun had lost its intensity. School would start in late August, but until then, we were in our own little world where gluten was not an issue. We ate the majority of our meals at home and spent our free time at the barn.

Sydney's riding progressed, and I continued giving the girls frequent lessons. I gradually took the horses off the lunge line and let the girls ride freely in the ring. While Foxie was completely reliable on the ground and on the lunge line, she had another side to her.

One day, I was standing in the middle of the ring calling out instructions to Sydney and Lauren-Kate. Now that it was summer, the sun was still high in the sky during the late afternoon. Heat pressed on my back and moisture gathered under my arms. Foxie's neck was damp with sweat, and her trot had a little more spunk to it than usual. I asked the girls to do several transitions from walk to trot, trot to walk and halt to make sure Sydney maintained control of her horse. But the mare continued to be more energetic than normal. So, I insisted Sydney make her halt every ten steps.

I could tell my daughter was getting frustrated with the slow pace of the lesson. "When Foxie speeds up," I instructed, "you have to remind her that you're in charge."

Without any warning, Foxie shied, and her hindquarters gathered underneath her. The sudden movement caused Sydney to lose her stirrups and slip to the right. Foxie took off at a gallop, racing toward the opposite end of the ring. My breath caught in my chest, and I imagined Sydney sliding off and rolling on the hard ground. She had a helmet on, but a fall would hurt and certainly scare her.

"Straighten up and tighten your reins!" I called out. Sydney clung to Foxie like a burr, grabbing a piece of the mare's mane and righting herself. Instinctively, I glanced over to make sure the gate to the big pasture was closed. If Foxie escaped the ring there was no telling how far she'd run. Thankfully, the gate was closed.

"Turn her into the fence to stop her!" I yelled. Those few seconds before Sydney managed to turn Foxie felt like an eternity. Finally, she stopped the mare, and Foxie stood with her flanks quivering.

I rushed over to Sydney who was clearly shaken. Her cheeks were flushed and a bead of sweat ran down the side of her face. "You did great, Sweetie. I can't believe you hung on." Inside, my mind was spinning. I needed to calm my daughter and give her confidence that she could handle situations like this. Yet, at the same time, I wondered how safe it was for her to ride Foxie.

Lauren-Kate walked Misty over to where Sydney and Foxie were standing. "I didn't think we were ready to canter yet; but I guess Foxie didn't know that," she said. Her wry comment broke the tension and made Sydney smile.

Over the next two weeks, I rode Foxie several times, hoping to nip this behavior in the bud. But when Foxie took off with Sydney a second time, I realized this tendency to take off was probably why Foxie was no longer a therapy horse. She had learned that she could take advantage of inexperienced riders.

My daughter's interest in riding started to wane. I explained to her my assessment of Foxie, that her behavior was not something that could be easily fixed. I told her we should consider selling Foxie and searching for a safer horse.

But Sydney would have none of it. She still spent her afternoons at the barn brushing Foxie and braiding her mane. She also cleaned her stall and gave her fresh shavings, scrubbed her water bucket and fed her every evening.

"We can't sell her, Mom. I love her."

"I'm not sure Foxie is the right horse for you," I responded. "I want you to be able to ride. You're spending so much time taking care of her. It's a lot of work. You should at least get the benefit of riding."

"I'll learn to control her. I will. She's my Foxie," she answered.

Sydney was tenderhearted, but she had a will of steel. I could tell she had her mind set and would do anything to keep her horse. But how could a beginner rider gain the experience to control a horse like Foxie?

Eventually, I came up with a plan. It wasn't foolproof, but it was something we could try. A friend of a friend was looking for a temporary home for a mare named April who had been in a lesson program. April was a little smaller than Foxie and, as her owner said, she had more "whoa" than "go," so she was perfect for a beginner rider. If Sydney could ride April regularly for six months, there was a good chance she'd develop a strong enough seat and the confidence to keep Foxie under control if she tried to take off. I talked with Sydney about this idea, and she agreed to give April a try. In the meantime, I would continue riding Foxie to give her some additional training. Smokey would have to go home, to Sydney's chagrin. She had been using him to give pony rides to children in our church. Sydney begged to keep Smokey, but three horses was already more than I had bargained for, and four was out of the question.

April arrived at the farm in the beginning of August. Despite the heat, Sydney spent the three weeks before school riding April every chance she could. Within two months, Sydney learned to walk, trot and canter on April. She even started jumping her over cross rails.

Sydney eased into school and her new schedule of studying and eating away from home as easily as she adjusted to riding April. My daughter was mature enough and established in her gluten-free ways to manage. She brought her lunch every day as did most of her friends, and she simply sat out when there was food in the classrooms. It wasn't pleasant for her to see classmates enjoying donuts, pancakes, pizza, or whatever the food du jour was. But she was used to saying "No, thanks. I'm allergic to gluten." Gradually, her friends and some of her teachers made the effort to provide gluten-free alternatives, which she didn't always eat, but she did appreciate their thoughtfulness.

For me, the biggest challenge turned out to be making lunches. I was used to providing three meals and snacks every day for her. But it was different having to think ahead and pack food that had to be kept cold or hot. Sandwiches—the typical lunch food—were something Sydney rarely ate. Unlike regular bread, the gluten-free kind came from the freezer section, and we kept it refrigerated, so it was cold and hard. At home for lunch, I usually gave my daughter leftovers from dinner that had to be reheated. While that worked at home, hot meals turned into lukewarm meals after hours in a thermos, and some of them became just plain unappealing. If Sydney didn't like what I packed, she couldn't stop at the vending machine for a snack. And there was never the option to send her to school with lunch money. As a noncook, I felt the strain and luxuriated in the freedom of non-school days when I didn't have to think ahead. Eventually, I fell into a routine of making big pots of spaghetti at night. If I didn't let Joel and Sydney have seconds, I could divide the leftovers into lots of lunches.

I became slightly more creative as time went on. Just slightly. And Sydney gradually took over the responsibility of making her own lunches. Sometimes she brought microwavable meals or leftovers from the weekend. She also packed fruit, crackers and other gluten-free convenience food.

In general, despite the challenge of making lunches, Sydney had plenty to eat and, most importantly, she didn't get sick. Yes, sometimes she yearned to indulge in the same snacks the other kids were eating. But not being able to eat them didn't pose any major problems.

Perhaps coming home to the barn and her friend Lauren-Kate, who was also gluten free, helped smooth the transition. As Sydney continued riding April, I wondered if my daughter's loyalties would shift. From Foxie to April, from horses to school activities. But she never wavered. Her goal was to ride Foxie and keep her under control. She kept that in the front of her mind. The traditional school schedule took up a lot more of her time than homeschooling, but Sydney was still always eager to come to the barn and spend time with Lauren-Kate and the horses.

After almost every lesson with April, she'd ask me, "Can I ride Foxie next time?" I wanted to be sure she was ready, so I waited. But Sydney kept pushing.

The day she got back on Foxie, two months shy of the six I had predicted she would need, I wasn't sure what to expect. As a mom, I wanted to keep my daughter safe and avoid any danger the same way I had tried to keep gluten out of her life. But just like with wheat exposures, I couldn't walk ahead of Sydney and clear the path of every possible hazard. And Sydney didn't want that from me. She had turned fourteen that fall, gone back to school, navigated the challenges of having celiac in a gluten-filled community and was growing into an independent young woman. Sydney was determined to ride her horse, to show me that she could do it, whether I was ready or not.

Sydney snapped the strap of her helmet under her chin and mounted Foxie. She walked her once around the ring and took off at a trot. "Keep your weight in your heels," I called after her. "And if you feel her speeding up, lean back and circle her."

"I know, Mom," said Sydney.

I thought she'd be content to take a short ride, to trot Foxie a few times around the ring and do more the next time. But Sydney asked if she could canter.

"Why don't we wait," I suggested.

"I can do it, Mom. She's being good."

I couldn't argue. Foxie was being a model horse, listening and responding to her rider's every move. But that didn't mean she wouldn't take off if given the chance. I watched her pale ears flick back and forth as Sydney talked to her.

"Okay," I said. "But let's keep her on a twenty-meter circle. If she speeds up, even a little bit, bring her right back to a trot."

Sydney nodded, and I watched the dapples on Foxie's belly glint in the sun. It was a warm fall day, and the sand in the ring created clouds of dust as Sydney circled one end of the ring at a trot. I saw her legs shift slightly, giving her horse the aids to the canter. Foxie's ears were up, and horse and rider worked in tandem, flowing into the gait like liquid. Sydney's face was a mask of concentration, but she moved comfortably in the saddle as if she was enjoying Foxie's smooth canter. After a couple of minutes, she brought Foxie back to a trot and then a walk, leaning over to pat her shoulder.

"I did it, Mom!" she called out as a smile spread across her face.

I let out the breath I'd been holding. "Yes, you did! I'm so proud of you." I didn't realize it at the time, but this was one of my lessons in letting go.

Eating Out

*O*ver time, because the transition to school was so seamless, I began to wonder if Sydney was becoming less sensitive to gluten. Could she be one of those rare people I'd read about who, with a slow, steady reintroduction of gluten, could eat wheat again? It seemed unlikely. Those cases were few and far between. Yet, during the past weeks and months, surely Sydney had come into contact with breadcrumbs from her friends' sandwiches. She'd managed to get through two years of school without a hint of nausea. Maybe, just maybe, she was outgrowing her severe sensitivity to gluten. Or was she bound to have another gluten exposure? Only time would tell.

Now that Sydney was a teenager, it had been both nerve wracking and a joy to see her caution around food settle down. She ate fast food at Chick Fil-A, pizzas at Mellow Mushroom and ventured into restaurants where the menus didn't explicitly say "gluten free," (although she was always careful to spell out her food needs to the wait staff). I couldn't help but think her body was adapting. We were both pretty sure she'd had some minor cross-contaminations without any serious consequences. Perhaps, even if she did have a full-on gluten exposure, it wouldn't be that bad.

As fate would have it, that exposure came on the heels of Hurricane Irma, just after school started in September of 2017. For several days we'd been watching the Weather Channel, praying for relatives who lived further south as the enormous storm—larger than the entire peninsula of Florida—devastated islands in the Caribbean and crept towards Miami and the Keys.

We were considered "in the cone," a scary designation given that twenty-eight years earlier Hurricane Hugo had ripped through Charlotte and our neck of the woods, upending huge oak trees and leaving most of the local residents without power for two weeks. As big as Hurricane Irma was, it seemed likely that most of the Southeast would be affected.

Even though I knew the news media was hyping up the danger, I made a list of storm preparations. We now had two horses at our barn—Foxie and Shady, Lauren-Kate's new horse. We relied on a well for their drinking water and our own. It was easy to fill up bottles of water for us, but horses drank a lot more than we did. If the power went out for any length of time, we'd have to haul thousands of pounds of water. So, I sent my husband out in search of a generator (just in case!), and I filled up every outside water tub in all the paddocks.

We filled up our cars with gas, and Sydney and I went shopping for gluten-free essentials, enough to get us through at least several days. I cleaned out our freezer to make space in case we needed to fill up bags of ice and use it as a large cooler. I also located our old propane camping stove in the garage.

Joel's parents were evacuated from Hilton Head Island and drove to our house. Joel's brother Bruce and his wife Kitty holed up in a shelter in Tampa with their three dogs as the hurricane track veered slightly west. I prayed for other friends, family members and cousins as the hurricane engulfed Florida.

Thankfully, Irma's bark was worse than her bite. At least for most of the people we knew. Yes, there was some damage and lots of debris everywhere. But our friends and family were safe. Amazingly, with cell phones, Facebook and Instagram, we were able to hear from people just prior to and immediately after the storm passed. My sister-in-law reported that their house still had power when she, Bruce and the dogs returned to it.

Our relief was palpable. But Irma, even though downgraded to a tropical storm, was still headed north. We were no longer in the cone, but rain was falling, and the wind was beginning to pick up in our part of the Carolinas.

Foxie and Shady rode out the worst of the weather in their stalls. I let them out for short bits so they wouldn't get too antsy. On Monday night, we went out to dinner to celebrate my mother-in-law's birthday. The outer bands of the storm passed over us as we drove to the restaurant.

Joel, Sydney and I had been to this restaurant a handful of times and had never had an issue with ordering gluten-free or dairy-free food. But the menu didn't explicitly state that any of the entrees were gluten free, so I felt it was important to be clear with the staff. They warned us that there was a chance of cross-contamination. Both Joel and Sydney rolled their eyes at me when I shared my concern.

A little over an hour later, we left the restaurant full and content and drove over to the yogurt store for birthday treats. I abstained, while Joel found a gluten-free, dairy-free option. Sydney had recently made the decision to add dairy back into her diet. She was willing to put up with some congestion and minor digestive issues if she could eat like her friends. I couldn't blame her. I knew being gluten free was hard enough. So, she enjoyed a cup of frozen yogurt.

That night the winds rose to twenty-five, maybe thirty miles per hour. I kept the horses in and closed the big barn doors to keep debris from blowing through the aisle.

The next morning, I woke up early to check on Foxie and Shady. Our driveway was littered with leaves and branches. From the mess in their stalls, it was obvious the horses had been nervous during the night. There had been hard rain, and probably they startled each time something fell on the tin roof of the barn. But thankfully, they were fine, and there was no major damage.

Joel's parents continued to watch the storm coverage and made the decision to try to return home the next day. Before they left, we planned one more meal out. Usually, I cooked at home, even when we had guests. It was just easier and safer. But I was tired, and Joel was eager to take us to the club, where he played golf and had served as president the previous year. The main dining room wasn't open, but the café, a casual snack bar in the tennis center was.

Before this summer, I could count the number of times our family had eaten out on two hands. So, for us to go out twice, back-to-back was really unusual! A part of me smiled, thinking of how I was returning to my old noncooking ways, now that Sydney was older and our concerns about gluten were diminishing. I daydreamed about going to the café on a weekly basis. The menu was small, but it touted gluten-free items, and we could wear jeans. A plus for both me and Sydney.

It was especially nice not to have to cook after living through the anxiety of watching Hurricane Irma for the past several days. Now that the worst of it had passed, and everyone we knew (including the horses) were safe, we could relax and enjoy an easy dinner.

Joel was excited for Sydney to try the gluten-free pizza. He had eaten it before, when the café had first opened, and he'd found it tasty. Mostly, though, he was pleased to show off his golf club to his parents, and he was proud that this little eatery was now serving food his family could eat.

None of us gave a thought to the horrible birthday pizza that had come from Joel's golf club many years earlier. Even if we had, I'm sure we would have waved off any concerns. This was a new café; gluten-free food was on the menu, not a special order. Plenty of other people had eaten here, and we'd not heard of any problems.

Joel's parents ordered their gluten-filled meal, while Joel and I ordered salads with grilled chicken. Sydney later told me she almost ordered a salad. But Joel had pointed to the pizza, declaring with a smile, "This is what you want!"

As we waited for the meal, Joel told us about the special pizza oven (approved by the board) at the café that cooked pizza in half the time. The manager stopped by our table to talk with Joel. My husband asked her why they no longer offered the gluten-free bread option with the BLT, and she said the kitchen was so small there was danger of cross-contamination. Perhaps that should have raised my antennae. But it didn't.

A few minutes later, our food appeared. Sydney's pizza was actually two small pizzas dripping with cheese.

Even though I was delighted with my plain salad topped with chicken, I couldn't help but notice how the mozzarella stretched into thin lines as my daughter lifted her first piece to her mouth. Was I envious? Maybe just a little. But I knew dairy didn't agree with me and, unlike Sydney, I wasn't surrounded by high school friends who ate it all day, so I let go of the idea of eating pizza, like the self-righteous mother I can be (when I must).

Joel, on the other hand, despite his own allergy to dairy, demanded she give him at least one slice. Sydney was happy to hand one over in exchange for a piece of chicken from his salad. Joel also eyed his father's meatball sub. Fortunately, it was too far away for him to reach.

As often happens, we began talking about food. "I could probably make you a gluten-free version of one of those at home," I said, pointing to Joel's father's plate.

"You could?" My husband's eyebrows lifted, and I could see I had fully attracted his attention.

"Sure. It would just take meatballs, some spaghetti sauce and a toasted gluten-free roll. The roll would be the hardest thing to find," I mused, wondering why I hadn't considered doing this before now. Maybe I could make one for Joel's birthday. December was a few months away. That would give me plenty of time to back out or for him to forget if I wasn't up to the task.

Sydney brought up the subject of her birthday cake. She asked if she could have "a really good one from the store."

I looked at her and pretended to cry. "You don't like my cakes?" I told her I'd be happy to buy her one from the store, if she could eat a normal cake. But a good gluten-free, dairy-free cake was outrageously expensive to order. I turned stern. "I'm not buying you a one-hundred-dollar cake."

"I want a cake with dairy in it," she whined.

"Dairy?" I said incredulously. Just because she was eating it, did she have to make her parents suffer—either from congestion and digestive issues if we ate a dairy-filled cake or from green-eyed envy as we watched her indulge?

"No, you can't have one with dairy," Joel joined in the conversation and put a stop to Sydney's dairy dreams. "Then I can't eat it."

"I don't think we can find a gluten-free Boston Crème Pie," I said. Boston Crème Pie had been a tradition in Joel's family, started by his grandmother who had lived in Boston and made delicious three-layer cakes for all his birthdays. It happened to be Sydney's current favorite.

"Well, I at least want one with carbs." I smiled thinking of the experiments I'd concocted over the years. Gluten-free, dairy-free, potato-free, low-carb cakes. I was happy to eat them because they were sweet. And Joel liked anything that was put in front of him. But to a normal kid, even one who is used to going gluten free, some of those cakes were just plain gross.

"I'll make you a cake with carbs," I conceded. "I can always use a box mix." I was thankful that over the years, it had become much easier to find gluten-free cake mixes. They were even available in regular grocery stores now.

After the meal, we hugged Sydney's grandparents and said goodbye. They would be leaving for home, hoping to avoid the worst of the returning evacuation traffic. I let out a sigh and said a small prayer that we could all return to our normal lives.

As we drove home, I spotted Foxie grazing in the big pasture. The horses were safe and out again after days of grey rain and strong winds. It felt as if they were a symbol of peace. Sunny, our golden retriever, greeted us at the door, and Joel and I decided to take her for a walk since she'd been inside more than usual over the past few days.

Sydney headed inside to finish up her homework. School had just started, and today was the first day of real homework. Tomorrow she had a test on an eight-hundred-page book she'd been assigned over the summer.

When Joel and I came back from walking the dog, we straightened up the kitchen, and I began stowing the empty bottles we'd put out on our telephone table in case we needed to fill them with water. I heard Sydney in her room FaceTiming one of her friends.

A few minutes later, she opened the door to her room and went into the bathroom.

When Sydney walked into the kitchen, she told me, "I just threw up." Her face was a mask of misery.

In that split second everything shifted. "The pizza?" I asked.

Sydney nodded, and I knew. But maybe, just maybe she was just tired. Maybe this was one of those typical sick feelings, the kind that passes, or the kind that passes after you throw up once. Or, if this was due to gluten, maybe she could handle it better now. She was older, stronger. Surely, she'd had exposures recently and been able to fend off feeling sick.

I followed Sydney into the bathroom.

"It's happening again. I can feel it," she said, putting her hand to her forehead. "Why?"

"Oh, Sweetie. I'm so sorry." I rubbed her back tentatively, wanting to take the horrible feeling of nausea away, but knowing, as a teenager, she didn't want me babying her.

"Why did I have to eat that pizza?" she moaned.

"It's not your fault. We didn't know." She leaned over the sink and the contents of her stomach splashed out.

I wet a cloth and handed it to Sydney. She wiped her face and asked for water. I couldn't help but remember the times we'd been in this same bathroom for hours. How she'd sobbed, saying "My tummy hurts," as she swayed against me. She still wanted and needed comfort. But I couldn't hold her on my lap the way I did then.

I checked my watch. Maybe, this would be over soon. In the past she'd thrown up every couple of minutes for a span of two hours until every last bit of gluten was purged from her system. Five minutes passed and ten.

At the fifteen-minute mark, she began holding her stomach again. "I feel it," she said. "Why is this happening? It can't happen. I've got a test tomorrow. I've got homework. If this was the middle of the year, I could skip a day. But school just started. I can't miss tomorrow." She spoke as if her words could change the inevitable.

I hoped against hope that her body could handle it better. That somehow this cycle of purging would not progress on its typical course. I didn't want that for her. "Oh, God, please make it stop!" I prayed silently.

But it didn't. Despite the first fifteen-minute window, each period of getting sick got closer and closer together, until she was throwing up every two minutes. At one point, she worried she might pass out, and I urged her to lie down on the couch. I brought out a big bowl and a wet washcloth.

All I could do was sit with her and watch her agony. Each time Sydney bent her head over the bowl, I'd empty it in the toilet, wash it out and refill her glass of water. As time went on, her stomach hurt more and more. I worried that with the intensity of her throwing up, her stomach might start bleeding.

Eventually, after two hours of the same awful cycle, the yellow bile began to come up. The only positive (if you could call it that) was that I knew enough from past experience to suggest that she drink water so that her body would have something to expel. Sydney was bigger and stronger, not the tiny waif who had seemed impossibly small and frail all those years ago. But her strength might make her body fight even harder. At times she had dry heaves, and her face had gone so pale.

I encouraged her to lie back against the pillows, to close her eyes and allow herself to fall asleep. During previous episodes like this, sleep had been the only thing that stopped the horrible sequence of vomiting. At one point, she murmured, "I can't sleep. I have work to do." And I could see her fighting.

"Your body needs rest," I said gently. "We'll figure out what to do in the morning."

"I'm going to school," she said stoically. "I can't miss."

As she continued getting sick, she gradually let go of the fight. She dozed on the couch for a few minutes, and I suggested she get in bed. Once asleep, hopefully, the nausea would begin to subside.

She stumbled towards her room, and I followed her with the bowl, the damp washcloth and a glass of water. She got into bed and after a few minutes vomited again.

After cleaning herself up, she laid back against her pillow and said, "I'll be fine."

"Are you sure?"

"Bye, Mom." My teenager was back. I took a deep breath and stepped out of her room.

The next morning, I heard her get up early and pour herself a bowl of cereal. I knew she'd be hungry after going through the night with nothing in her stomach. I also knew she wanted to test herself to see if she could keep food down. She could, though she didn't have much appetite. And she was going to school.

In the kitchen, her face looked drawn. She picked at the scrambled eggs Joel had made for her.

"You don't have to eat those, honey," I said.

She worried that she'd be starving by midmorning, so I suggested she bring an extra snack. When Sydney set her mind to something there was no changing it, so I didn't try to talk her out of going to school. But I did ask her to call me if she didn't feel well. I didn't expect to get a call.

Joel drove Sydney to school that morning and had plans to play golf. He said as soon as he was done, he would stop by the café and talk to the staff about the pizza. It obviously wasn't his fault, but I knew he felt bad and wanted to understand what had gone wrong.

That afternoon, Sydney came home from school, lay down on her bed and fell asleep. Through sheer determination, she'd made it through the day. But she had nothing left.

When Joel got home, he told me about his return visit to the café. Both the manager and waitress from the night before were on duty.

I had questions: What were the ingredients in the crust? And the sauce? Was the pizza cooked on a pan or directly on the rack where other gluten crusts had been laid? Was it possible the pan had been dusted with regular flour?

Not surprisingly, neither the manager nor the staff admitted to any mistakes or cross-contamination issues. Apparently, every time anyone ordered a gluten-free pizza, the staff went through a particular routine. Last night, the waitress performed the routine as she usually did.

I couldn't help but be suspicious. Something had gone wrong. Our daughter had endured a horrendous evening. She didn't ask to be poisoned. She had simply trusted. The menu said "gluten free" in black and white, and the pizza wasn't!

Joel was less emotional and resigned to believing what he was told. "The only thing they could come up with was that they just started ordering their gluten-free dough from another bakery, and maybe it's not safe," he said.

"Or maybe they used the wrong dough on Sydney's pizza." I wanted to find the culprit, blame someone. But, of course, this was one of those situations where we would not learn the answer.

I looked up the name of the "new dough" online, and it had a gluten-free label. It should have been fine. Maybe it was, and maybe it wasn't. Maybe the waitstaff made a mistake. Maybe they didn't. All I knew for sure was that my daughter had paid a dear price.

Later, after Sydney woke up and joined us for dinner, Joel told her what he'd learned from the manager. Like me, she was sorry not to have conclusive evidence of a mistake. But she accepted Joel's explanation better than I did. Maybe she was just tired, or maybe she knew it wasn't worth the energy to fight an invisible foe. Instead, she declared emphatically: "I will never eat pizza at the club again. Ever!"

Letting Go (Older Teenager)

*D*espite her experience at the café, Sydney was growing and maturing, expanding her boundaries and making her own choices and decisions around food. She had a short list of favorite restaurants—Chick Fil-A and P.F. Chang's—she visited regularly. There were many more such as Mellow Mushroom, Boston Market and Carrabba's where she ate, and our family was able to dine safely.

As the parent of an older teenager, my services as a cook were suddenly needed less frequently. I could see a time in the not-too-distant future when I could hang up my apron. I would not return to the sandwiches and subs of old. But, in a sense, it felt as if I was coming full circle.

Trips became so much easier. My daughter was taking responsibility for her own food. I still packed a cooler, but I no longer had to think ahead about every meal. I had learned to bring celery and sliced cucumbers for myself and carrots and almonds for my husband to snack on in the car, so we didn't have to survive on gas-station fare, which still had a long way to go when it came to gluten-free options. If we were hungry, we could always grab a pack or two of roasted almonds or other nuts. No longer did I pack fruit, chips, gluten-free bars and other assorted snacks for Sydney. On the road, she preferred to eat at fast-food restaurants, go to the grocery store or "figure it out" herself.

Vacations became less work for me since I did not have to cook every meal. On our last trip to the mountains, for instance, Sydney ordered lunch at Chick-Fil-A. For dinner, Joel and Sydney indulged in gluten-free pizza while I had a salad with grilled chicken and bacon. We all declared that our food was delicious!

I learned, though, that my digestive system appreciated my caution. I slept better at night (literally) when I carried my own pack of chicken (which I knew was gluten free) rather than took a chance at a restaurant. While some cooks and eating establishments were safe, many were not. Even when they tried to be conscientious, their knowledge was simply limited. I mean how many people have spent the last ten years studying where gluten might be hiding and the dangers it posed? You only did that if you *had* to!

On that same trip to the mountains, I was enjoying *not* being the overly crazed, gluten-intolerant patron at a chain restaurant so much that I made a mistake with my salad. Either the chicken had been processed with wheat or the bacon had been cross-contaminated. I found this out when I went to bed and was unable to sleep through the night (even though I had taken an intense five-mile hike that day). My body was tired, but something deep inside my system was thrumming (no doubt working to clear itself of gluten). I lay there with my eyes closed knowing that at best I'd get a few interrupted periods of sleep during the night. And in the wee hours way past midnight, I felt that old sensation of pain in my gut. Rather than stress over it, I chalked it up to experience.

Next time, I would remember my GlutenEase (a supplement designed to help clear gluten from the system) or bring my baggie of chicken. I knew that the worst symptoms would subside after three days, and I would gradually be able to sleep through the night again. I was fortunate that I did not react as severely as Sydney did with a gluten exposure, and I was thankful that both she and Joel were fine after eating their dinner.

Despite the gluten incident, I still felt a growing sense of freedom. I knew how to nourish myself and my family. My daughter was taking responsibility for her own food choices. We could do things we used to be afraid to consider. We were traveling more, beginning to imagine and plan trips to more far-flung places like California and Hawaii, even Europe. Some of it was experience. We had been there and paid the price. I could prepare a week's worth of food in my sleep (almost), we could scour the internet for gluten-free restaurants and take chances if we chose. Most grocery stores now, even non-specialty ones, carried enough gluten-free food that we could survive. Each day was an adventure, rather than a scary walk through a gluten-filled world.

Grandparents

*O*n a recent trip to visit Joel's parents, I had an interesting conversation with them about celiac disease. Sydney and I were sitting around the kitchen table eating breakfast with her grandparents. Joel had gone to meet his brother for a round of golf.

I brought up the fact that I was writing a memoir about how our family had gone gluten free, and I wanted to get their perspective on what it was like having a granddaughter who had celiac disease.

I was surprised at Joel's father Anton's response. "It's been a real hardship for us," he pronounced. In the middle of the table was a box of gluten-filled cookies he'd purchased for his grandkids. Of course, Sydney could not eat them.

I looked at Anton in surprise, waiting for him to continue. He stirred blueberries into his oatmeal. "Her celiac makes it tough on us."

I raised my eyebrows. "Really?"

"I can't even make oatmeal for her. I'd like to be able to treat my granddaughter," he said.

"Well, how do you think it feels to Sydney?" I countered. "Everybody else gets to eat whatever they want, and Sydney (not to mention her parents) can only have certain things."

"I know. We'd like to take you all out to eat. But we have to worry about everything being gluten free," he said.

"I want to give Sydney these cookies." Anton grabbed the package in front of him. "But I can't." This was the same man who went to three grocery stores looking for gluten-free/dairy-free ice cream for Sydney.

I was used to bringing coolers of food to Joel's parents' house and making most of our own meals. So, I didn't have a lot of empathy for Anton. I mean, in my mind, we were the ones who were suffering. Not him. But he did bring up a good point. I'd never thought about how grandparents like to spoil their grandkids. That certainly wasn't easy to do in Sydney's case.

Even going out to eat was a challenge. There were very few restaurants that offered gluten-free menus, and of those, not all were considered safe. Sydney's grandparents would have been overjoyed if they could take us out to dinner every night.

"I wish Sydney could eat *my* cookies," said Sally.

Sydney glanced up from her bowl of Rice Chex as I sighed. "I wish she could too."

Joel's mother was used to baking her special Swedish Spritz cookies and giving a tin of them to each of her sons at Christmas. It was something they had grown up with and looked forward to each Christmas. Heck, so did I. Those cookies were light and buttery and melted in our mouths. After we went gluten free, we could no longer accept her gift of cookies. They were too much of a temptation for Joel. Even though he was allergic to gluten, he couldn't stop himself from eating his mother's Spritz when they were under his nose.

Sally also made delicious Swedish meatballs during holidays that suddenly were off-limits to us. For many years, she'd send a container of meatballs home with us or bring one when she and Anton visited. She was a wonderful cook, and sharing her food was one of the ways she showed her love. And it had always been appreciated.

After our family stopped eating gluten, I asked her for her recipe, and I was able to make a pretty good facsimile of the meatballs. But I didn't even try to replicate the Spritz. I knew they were beyond my skill set. From my other cookie-baking fails, I'd learned that some things are just not the same without gluten.

Of course, the selfish part of me wondered, why couldn't Sally make some of her meals gluten free? It was not that hard to substitute a few ingredients. I knew that both Sally and Anton were deeply concerned about Sydney's health. They'd had first-hand experience with the dangers of a gluten exposure after being present at Sydney's tenth birthday party. Maybe Sally didn't want to take the chance of making a mistake. Or, maybe, like most other people we'd met, until you've been the one not eating gluten, it's hard (possibly even overwhelming) to try to meet someone else's food requirements.

I thought about my parents and wondered how they would have responded to Sydney's celiac disease and our gluten-free lifestyle. Like Anton, my father (who died the year before Sydney was born) had enjoyed dispensing treats. He would have offered Sydney candy from the stash he kept in his pockets. She would have learned quickly to accept it, but not necessarily eat it, if she didn't trust the ingredients. Yet my father would have continually handed it out.

Eventually, after intense education and strict instruction (by me), my father would have found one or two safe treats Sydney could enjoy. He would have purchased those things for her by the bushel.

If my mom hadn't had Alzheimer's disease, I imagine she would have gone out of her way to make something special for Sydney. Chocolate chip cookies or cake or fudge. Or if she didn't trust herself to not contaminate her granddaughter in the baking process, she would have kept her eye out (as Joel's mother often did) for stores that carry gluten-free baked goods. My mom would have delighted in presenting Sydney with a tissue-wrapped Danish or a box of donuts. If she couldn't find a store, my mother would have sought out an online specialty shop and ordered a gift-wrapped container of gluten-free sweets for Sydney, no matter the cost. At least that's what I like to think she would have done.

Many people in Sydney's life (including her grandparents, aunts, uncles, cousins and friends) have gone above and beyond, ordered the specialty box of gluten-free goodies (even a six-month supply!), baked a delicious gluten-free cake or a platter of brownies or cookies, picked up a box of gluten-free cupcakes or donuts, searched the supermarket freezers for the brand of ice cream Sydney can eat, treated us to meals at restaurants that offer gluten-free fare. These thoughtful, generous souls have done much to alleviate the pain of "missing out."

Prom

*I*t was a muggy spring Saturday, and Sydney was up and out of the house by midmorning in order to get her nails and hair done. She had found a prom dress at the mall. It had a dark blue bodice trimmed with silver applique and a floor-length, white tulle skirt. In the dressing room, as she kicked off her tennis shoes and shorts and pulled up the gown, my eyes had filled with tears because she looked like a princess.

After a few passing showers, the weather cleared, and Sydney's date, who was a friend, came to the house. Joel and I took photos as they exchanged flowers. We followed them to one of their friends' houses where a group of kids were meeting, and parents were invited to take photos for an hour before the limo came to pick them up and drive them to the Speedway Club. The outdoor photos were spectacular against a background of green grass, blossoming trees and spring flowers. The girls were decked out in an array of colorful gowns, the guys handsome in their black suits and tuxes. Sydney was full of joy, surrounded by her friends and anticipating a fun night ahead. Joel and I had driven separately so we could drop off Sydney's car at another friend's house. There would be an afterparty and most of the girls in her class would spend the night together there.

Prom was a marker in their lives, and for me it held extra significance. It was evidence that Sydney had not only survived the transition to traditional school, but she was thriving, enjoying a full life

179

with friends and social activities. She was on the Prom Committee with her classmates, and they had chosen a unique location, the Speedway Club, part of the Charlotte Motor Speedway, a place where there would be dinner and dancing; part of the meal—the meat and the veggies—would be gluten free, so that Sydney could eat without worrying. One of the moms even picked up gluten-free cupcakes for dessert.

We joined the other parents and followed the limo to the Speedway where the professional photographer was taking more photos. The entrance to the club was a whirl of pastel and jewel-colored gowns. Clumps of guys posed together as girls hugged each other and took pictures with their phones. Each class lined up for more photos. The backdrop was a striking, edgy contrast to the peaceful backyard we had just left. Steps led up to a tall, glass building which overlooked a brightly colored amusement park on the other side of the road, complete with a Ferris wheel. It felt like a metaphor for this stage in Sydney's life. She was leaving childhood behind and was on the brink of a new stage of independence. I took more photos of Sydney with her friends, hoping to capture her sense of excitement and joy.

After a little while, a couple of teachers ushered the students toward Smith Tower, the building that held the Speedway Club. Joel and I turned to leave and ran into some parents we knew. They were going to follow the kids and look at the decorated dinner and dance floor and invited us to join them. I didn't want to horn in on Sydney's evening, but I couldn't resist taking a peek.

We followed at a reasonable distance, waiting until Sydney and her date had left the lobby, then we took the elevator up to the club floor. The doors opened onto a magical setting. To one side was a staircase with luminaries on each step, and the room behind it was aglow with twinkling fairy lights.

I could imagine Sydney eating and dancing, posing for more photos, smiling and laughing. The other side of the elevator opened into the viewing area for races. There were rows of folding seats and a large plexiglass wall where race fans could watch cars circling the track. There were no races that night, but I made Joel sit with me for a moment so I could imagine what it would be like watching such speed as engine exhaust tickled my nose.

I also thought of my daughter racing towards graduation and her future. I was thankful we could press pause on this special evening. As Joel and I headed home, we felt a sense of ease knowing that for this night, Sydney was safely ensconced in her high school world, surrounded by friends and prom festivities.

At 11:05 p.m., my phone rang. I recognized the name immediately, and the hair on the back of my neck stood up. It was a friend, one of the prom chaperones. "I'm so sorry, Ann. But Sydney's sick. She says she thinks she might have had some gluten. She's okay, but she wants to go home."

"Oh, nooo!" I put my hand to my chest, picturing Sydney throwing up in her beautiful prom dress. My friend said kids were just starting to leave for the afterparty, but some of them were staying to clean up, and she would stay as well. I told her I would send Joel.

My husband had fallen asleep early, but he jumped up when he heard his name. "What's going on?"

"Gluten," I said, and his face clouded over. I told him where to pick up Sydney.

When he left, the phone rang again. This time it was Sydney.

"Oh, Sweetie, I'm so sorry," I said. "Are you okay?"

"I feel terrible," she said. "But I made it through most of the night. I was having so much fun." She described how she started feeling bad a couple hours after eating, and she went into the bathroom. Some of the girls followed to check on her. They told her that maybe it was just the heat and that she'd feel better soon. Sydney knew it was most likely gluten, but their words encouraged her enough to go back and try to dance again. She had only thrown up once and was feeling better, so maybe she'd be okay. But after the last dance, she knew. She said she barely made it back to the bathroom in time.

I told her Dad was on his way, then I asked, "What did you eat?"

"I just had a little bit of meat and the veggies, and the cupcakes were so good! Everything was supposed to be gluten free. And now I have to miss the afterparty."

"Oh, honey, I know. I'm so sorry."

When Sydney and Joel got home, she went straight to the bathroom. Despite her pale complexion, she still looked lovely—her hair held its curl from earlier, her makeup made her brown eyes stand out. She could have been Cinderella. After she threw up, I wiped her face with a damp washcloth, eased her out of her dress and set her up on the couch with a plastic bowl.

In between trips to the bathroom, she filled me in on the details of the night. She and her date were having a great time. They danced to almost every song. My heart lifted a little as I heard the remnants of joy in her voice. She knew she probably should have double-checked with the chef about the food. But there was a long line, and she didn't want to be disruptive. The meal tasted good. But there was a sauce on the meat. We decided maybe that was the culprit. She was grateful she didn't start feeling bad until the very end. At least she got to enjoy most of the night.

Sydney chattered after each bout of throwing up. The excitement of the night was clearly still with her. I was amazed at her cheerfulness in the midst of a beautiful evening gone awry. And I was grateful for her sweet friends and the kind moms who called and texted to check on her. Sydney's sudden illness had been a shock to them. Most of them knew about her celiac disease, but they had never witnessed the aftereffects of a gluten exposure. Seeing this night end so drastically concerned them all.

While I hated that she had to go through this, and I was especially sad that her prom night was marred, I couldn't help but see the blessing in having her friends experience a little bit of her reality. Sydney had never been one to bring attention to her condition. But perhaps this incident would open a door which would allow her friends to understand and support her in new ways.

Sydney survived the next few hours of continuous vomiting. Her face had a grey tint as she held her stomach and pressed her hand to her head, closing her eyes. I gave her sips of water and watched as the bile eventually rose and spilled from her throat into the toilet. Still, during moments when she had a little bit of energy, she told stories about the limo ride and asked me to send her the photos I had taken.

The next couple of days were rough, as they usually are after a gluten exposure. Sydney spent most of Sunday in bed recovering from a headache, abdominal pain, dehydration and the severe inflammation in her digestive tract. Several of the moms continued to check in, asking how Sydney was doing. Joel, Sydney and I agreed it wasn't worth investigating the exposure and pursuing the issue. It was highly unlikely she'd ever return to the Speedway Club, and if she did, she certainly wouldn't eat there. But I was happy to share Sydney's sweet sentiment that lasted after the difficult weekend: "Mom, even though I got sick, I'm so glad I was able to enjoy most of the night."

Prom did turn out to be a marker in Sydney's life. But it wasn't the one I expected. Instead of the storybook evening I had imagined, the night had ended in disaster. But I was struck by Sydney's resilience. Not only was she able to join in on activities in a gluten-filled world, but when things went wrong, she could still find a way to thrive and appreciate the blessings.

College Tours

*A*t the time of Sydney's diagnosis, visiting colleges felt so far in the future I could hardly imagine it. But when I *had* thought about it, given my desire to keep my daughter safe and healthy, it made me cringe. How many colleges would offer gluten-free dining? And if they did, would it *really* be gluten-free, or would there be cross-contamination? Would Sydney be miles away from us suffering from a relentless, debilitating cycle of nausea and vomiting? Survival! That was number one in my mind.

And a close second was my daughter's social life. I didn't want Sydney to be segregated, unable to participate in the typical college rituals—campus functions involving food, late-night pizza and popcorn, outings with friends to local restaurants. Food was a part of life at home or at college, and I wanted her to be able to enjoy it all. Having to turn down food or pack her own would not be the same. Would she be able to eat in the dining hall with her friends or simply have to watch while they enjoyed all the menu items she couldn't have?

Over the years, my worries gradually lessened as eating gluten free became a way of life for all of us. As a high schooler, Sydney had moved to being cautiously adventurous in her eating. She embraced the opportunity to go out to eat and felt confident that she could find safe foods on the menu. She was also wise enough to know that if the waiter or waitress looked at her quizzically when she asked about gluten-free food that she should be extra careful. If her salad arrived with breadcrumbs on it, she asked for another and didn't try to eat around the crumbs. She had learned through experience how to take care of and speak up for herself.

Safe eating was important to Sydney, but she was growing into a young adult who made her own choices and was responsible for the outcome of those choices. As we visited colleges, we would be invited to have meals at various dining halls. I would have to learn to sit back and watch as we entered each venue. It would be up to her to ask questions, check out the menu and see how comfortable she felt. We would also drive around each college town and look at the eating establishments. Would there be a favorite restaurant that offered gluten-free food? I had no idea.

What I did know was that gluten-free dining was not the most important thing on Sydney's list. She would be looking at *all* the factors of college life (campus size, college personality, academics, sports, etc.) and weighing what was most important to her. What she decided and how she handled the food situation would also be up to her. It wouldn't be simple, but I trusted she could handle it.

By the beginning of 2020, Sydney had narrowed down the list of colleges she was interested in to two and was leaning strongly towards one—a small private school in the Charlotte area. Both schools were excellent choices, though neither appeared to have outstanding gluten-free dining options. At least they had not been named to any Top Ten U.S. Gluten-free College List. Out of curiosity, I periodically researched these lists. The only North Carolina college that consistently showed up was North Carolina State University, which I had encouraged Sydney to check out. But neither the size nor the location appealed to her. So, I had to drop it.

The college Sydney was interested in hosted a Scholarship Weekend in January, and she was one of dozens of students invited to participate. Parents were also encouraged to attend, so Joel and I made plans to spend the day on campus with her. In my mind, this was a great opportunity to scope out the dining options. Sydney was perfectly capable of sleuthing herself, but she wasn't driven like I was. So, I figured it couldn't hurt for there to be a second pair of eyes.

On Saturday morning, the three of us arrived a few minutes before the first session. We congregated with a few other families from Sydney's high school, standing near the continental breakfast table, I perused the choices. Serving platters overflowed with muffins and mouth-watering pastries. But nothing was gluten free. Sydney was used to skipping breakfast, so she ambled past the food without giving it a glance.

Our family attended the welcome speech from the president together, then we split up. Sydney joined other students for group activities and interviews while Joel and I heard a financial aid talk and a panel of parents and students discussing various aspects of student life. We would meet up with Sydney for lunch.

Joel and I arrived in the dining hall first. It was noisy and chaotic, filled with college and high school students, parents, admissions staff and professors. Various stations were set up cafeteria style, and the aromas of pizza, hamburgers, chicken and fresh-baked bread drifted from behind clear partitions.

Joel grabbed a flyer near a cashier and scanned it for gluten-free options while I walked from station to station to see what might be possible to eat. Nothing appeared to be labeled gluten free. I could feel my anxiety rising as I imagined Sydney struggling to find sustenance here.

We asked an elderly cashier if she could tell us where the gluten-free food was. The woman studied us for a moment before replying. "There's a market in the back." She pointed over her shoulder. "They have salads, soups and sandwiches. You should be able to find something there."

Hopeful, Joel and I shimmied through the crowds of people and made our way to "the market." It appeared to be a deli. Joel stood in line while I took a lap around the soup and salad bar. It had the usual fare—containers of lettuce, dressing and various vegetable toppings. There were two pots of warm soup.

I joined Joel at the front of the line, whispering my findings to him.

"What's gluten free?" Joel asked the cashier, who looked up and called to another worker who was preparing a sandwich. He repeated Joel's question.

I raised my eyebrows at Joel with a "This does not look promising look." The second worker responded: "The roasted turkey is gluten free, and we've got gluten-free bread. Also, the salad bar."

"What about the soups?" I asked. Sydney rarely ate soup, but if this was all they had, maybe she would learn.

"The lentil soup is gluten free. But the chicken soup has noodles in it."

Oh. I felt my stomach sinking. Lentil soup was not going to cut it. I had been hoping for clearly labeled meals: gluten-free pizza, pasta, chicken, hamburgers. Food that college students enjoyed. Not slices of turkey in between two pieces of dry, gluten-free bread. The salad bar was something. But lettuce, tomatoes, cucumbers and carrots would only go so far in filling up Sydney.

I remembered my own days at the college dining hall. The meals were hot, and I had choices of chicken, lasagna, meatloaf or spaghetti. Even if I didn't care for what was offered, I could always find something to fill up on. What would Sydney do on days when she had exams or a paper to write, and she and her friends made their way to the dining hall? Would she have to watch her friends select meals from a bountiful menu while she nibbled on a salad and a cold turkey sandwich? I sighed deeply.

My phone vibrated in my pocket. It was Sydney asking where we were. I texted her back and she told me where I could find her. I told Joel, who was asking for condiments for his sandwich, that I was going to meet her.

Erasing the frustration from my face, I made my way back to the front of the dining hall. It was less crowded now as many of the students and parents had found their way to a food station or were sitting down to eat. I told Sydney where her dad was and made light of the trouble we'd had in finding *anything* gluten free. Anxiety was rumbling around inside me. This was Sydney's top choice of colleges, and I didn't want my reaction to the food situation spoiling her visit. At least she was familiar with the city of Charlotte, and there were several restaurants and fast-food establishments nearby that served gluten-free items. If she had to, she could leave campus for her meals. Of course, *that* wouldn't be ideal.

"What do you want to do?" I asked her.

"Let's just walk around and check out what they have," she said casually.

"Okay." I continued to bite back the stream of bad news her father and I had uncovered as we wandered around examining a few of the stations. I was excited to see a couple of purple tags that denoted gluten-free items and pointed them out. Upon closer inspection, we realized the tags were for things like cereal and bread. Well, at least she would be able to get breakfast here.

After coming up empty on actual lunch foods, I reminded Sydney of "the market" where Joel and I had been. Uninterested in leaving the central eating area, she said, "Let's just ask someone." We walked over to the end of the main cafeteria line and waited for a worker to come out of the kitchen. A woman carrying a stack of trays stepped out, and Sydney caught her attention.

"We both have an allergy to gluten," my daughter said. "Is there anything we can eat here?"

"Let me talk to the chef. I'll be right back."

A moment later, a man in a white apron and a baseball hat strode over. "Are you the ones who are gluten free?"

"Yes." We both nodded.

"I'm allergic to dairy as well," I added. If gluten-free food was scarce in the dining hall, why not make the challenge doubly hard? It would be a good test.

"How does chicken, vegetables and potatoes sound?" the man responded. "The vegetables and potatoes are steamed, and I can make the chicken in a separate pan."

"That sounds great," Sydney and I said in unison. A balloon of hope rose inside me.

"I'll be back in seven or eight minutes," the chef said. "Have a seat."

Sydney and I joined the other families in the dining area and found an empty table. I texted Joel to let him know where we were. A moment later, he showed up with his turkey sandwich and salad. Unaware of my resolution to not complain about the lack of gluten-free options, Joel began sharing the details of our earlier adventures.

"We had to go all the way to the back," he said. "There was gluten-free bread and gluten-free turkey. Not a lot to choose from."

"Only one of the soups was gluten free," I added. "But there was a salad bar." Now that Joel had started the conversation, I added my concerns. "I was worried we wouldn't find *anything*! Do you think you could survive off slices of cucumber?" I picked one off Joel's plate and popped it in my mouth.

"How are you going to eat if you go here, Sydney?" Joel asked. "I hope you like sandwiches."

Sydney looked amused at us. "You guys are over the top," she said. "You don't have to worry about me. I can manage."

A few moments later, the chef rushed towards our table with two plates of food. He set them in front of Sydney and me. The aroma of freshly cooked chicken, steamed asparagus and cut-up potatoes made my mouth water.

I raised my eyebrows. "It's gluten free and dairy free, right?" I asked just to be sure.

"Yes. Gluten free and dairy free," he repeated with authority. "Do you need anything else?"

I waited for Sydney to answer. "We're fine. This looks great!"

As he walked away, Sydney and I dug into our meal. The chicken was tender and tasty, the potatoes lightly seasoned and the asparagus was perfectly cooked.

"This is delicious!" Sydney said.

"It really is!" I said.

"Can I have some of your potatoes?" Sydney asked.

"Sure." I scooped them onto her plate, and she nudged some asparagus onto mine. "This is like a first-class restaurant. You get your food delivered and everything! I had no idea it would be this good!"

Sydney smiled and shook her head. "Mom, I told you, you worry too much."

After we ate, Sydney and I wandered around the dining hall. The students had thinned out. Without the long lines and the chaos of so many people in one place, Sydney pointed out various purple tags we had missed earlier. It was nice to see there more choices than Joel and I had originally thought. I also remembered the admissions counselor sharing that the college had a Registered Dietitian on staff who was happy to meet with students to discuss their nutrition needs. Sydney had asked me not to contact her. She would do that herself if she felt the need. My daughter was right. She would be fine. It was time for me to let go.

The Changes in Our Family

What started out as a journey to heal my daughter and understand celiac has ended up benefitting our entire family. When I look back, I find it incredible how much our lifestyle and habits have changed. Eating out is no longer a way of life, though we have come back around to enjoying it from time to time. No longer are we oblivious to our food choices—buying only what looks tasty and ignoring the ingredients. Each of us understands the clear connection between what we eat and how we feel.

I am amazed at how far I've come since I was a sugar-addicted kid who avoided green vegetables like the plague. Clearing gluten from my body was the first step in finding a way to eat that would support my health. Going gluten free helped me feel, for the first time in my life, that food was truly nourishing me rather than contributing to a general sense of malaise, and I began to feel free.

With years of experience and research under my belt, I have become the resident celiac expert in my home and among my community of friends. My husband relies on me to provide healthy food that will keep his golf game in shape for many years to come.

Joel still "cheats" on occasion, but even those instances have changed. He has gradually taken responsibility for his own health. He no longer indulges in gluten-filled treats when they are dangled in front of his nose, but instead, makes wiser choices such as occasional desserts made without wheat or a handful or two of tortilla chips rather than the whole bag. Gone are the days of the wheat-filled meatball subs!

Sydney, who was always more careful than Joel, trusts me to be the gluten gatekeeper to our pantry; she knows I won't let it sneak in. As a young adult, she is wise about her choices and makes her own decisions about what she eats. Her radar for gluten is finely tuned, and she has learned to speak up for herself. She still gets frustrated, as any normal human being would, when she is on the outside looking in, and her friends are enjoying food that she can't have. But I could not be more proud of the strong woman she is becoming as she navigates a wheat-filled world.

Friends who are considering going gluten free or simply have concerns about their diet and health often come to me asking questions. Even Joel shares the success of our gluten-free lifestyle with fellow golfers. Of course, neither of us have all the answers. But we can share what has worked for us and our family.

What a joy it is to wake up feeling good. My days of bloating, constipation, achiness, sleeplessness and mild depression are, for the most part, a thing of the past. Eliminating gluten, dairy and, to a large degree, sugar have given my digestive tract a chance to heal.

My own journey towards good health is a never ending one, and I'm grateful for the many doctors and alternative healthcare practitioners that I've had the privilege to work with and learn from. In addition to feeling better than I ever have, the greatest gift is seeing my daughter and husband healthy and thriving in their own passions and pursuits.

Epilogue

COVID-19

*I*n March of 2020, life as we knew it drastically shifted as fears about the deadly and rapidly spreading coronavirus swept across the U.S. and the world. Every day brought a host of changes. On Mar. 12th, Joel was planning to fly to Brooklyn for the Atlantic10 Men's Basketball Tournament and to attend a music concert with a friend. But within a couple of days, basketball tournaments across the country went from business as usual to being played with no fans to being cancelled. Fortunately, Joel didn't get on the plane or he might have been quarantined in New York due to an outbreak of the virus in New Rochelle, just a few miles from his hotel. By the end of the week, all NCAA, pro and high school sports were shut down.

Sydney's last quarter of high school was about to be upended. Rules were changing rapidly as each state's government made decisions about what was safe. Social gatherings were restricted to no more than one hundred, then fifty, then ten people. Colleges sent students home midsemester. Sydney's Spring Break was extended from one to two weeks, then we received word that her school would begin online classes. The governor announced that public schools would be closed until May 15th, and a "stay-at-home" order was issued for North Carolina.

Gradually, every outside event dropped off our calendars or transitioned to a virtual meeting. People began working from home, and all businesses, except those deemed essential, closed. Restaurants shut the doors to their dining rooms and offered only take-out meals. Going to the grocery store became an adventure as people donned masks and gloves to shop. Toilet paper became a hot commodity! And staples such as chicken, hamburger and broccoli were not always available. Fortunately, we were well stocked with gluten-free food, and these items did not seem to disappear from the shelves as fast as many traditional ones.

Plans for Sydney's mid-May graduation were put on hold, and college orientations switched from on-campus to virtual events. As a former homeschooler, Sydney slipped easily into the routine of doing her schoolwork at home. She picked up to-go meals at Chick-Fil-A and purchased boxes of gluten-free macaroni and cheese, cookies and brownie mixes to make at home.

We never could have foreseen such a change in our world. And the future is unknown. No one can predict if we'll be able to return to our old lives or if what's "normal" will change forever. Although on a much smaller scale, in some ways, this shift mirrors what happened to our family when we received Sydney's celiac diagnosis. The habits we had come to rely on around food were suddenly wiped out. Knowing we were able to manage this fundamental change and build a new way of eating from the ground up, even though it was full of challenges, gives me hope. Not only is my daughter resilient, but so is our family. We have all learned to give up things we love in order to embrace our own health and each other.

In this new world where COVID-19 exists, people are altering their patterns to support those who are most vulnerable in our society. Eating in restaurants, going out for movie nights, attending music concerts or sporting events are, for now, a thing of the past. Phone calls and virtual meetings are replacing face-to-face visits. Church services are streamed live over the internet. Maybe hardest of all is not being able to hug family and friends or visit elderly loved ones in care communities. Yet, we are finding ways to express our feelings, pull together, support and nourish one another.

At a tender age, celiac disease taught Sydney to let go of what was harmful to her. At the time, it didn't seem fair. Why should she have to sacrifice when others around her could eat what they wanted? Now, as a young adult, my daughter is equipped in a unique way to face our rapidly changing world. I trust Sydney has the wisdom and fortitude to traverse the trials that lie ahead and quietly lead the way towards a healthy future for herself and others.

The End

Notes

Prologue

1. Celiac Disease Foundation, "What is Celiac Disease?" and "Symptoms of Celiac Disease." 1998-2020. https://celiac.org/.

Chapter 1: My History

2. Mayo Clinic, "Celiac disease: Symptoms & causes." 1998-2020. https://www.mayoclinic.org/diseases-conditions/celiac-disease/symptoms-causes/syc-20352220.

Chapter 16: My GF Journey

3. Justin Hollon, Elaine Leonard Puppa, Bruce Greenwald, Eric Goldberg, Anthony Guerrerio and Alessio Fasano, "Effect of Gliadin on Permeability of Intestinal Biopsy Explants from Celiac Disease Patients and Patients with Non-Celiac Gluten Sensitivity," *Nutrients,* Feb. 27, 2015. https://doi.org/10.3390/nu7031565.

Acknowledgments

Our family's gluten-free journey has spanned almost two decades and will no doubt continue for many more. But the first years were the hardest, and I am more than grateful to the people who helped us along the way and those who supported the writing of this book.

I'm grateful to Deb Waldron, M.S., R.D., Gilda Morina Syverson and Anthony Abbott for your beautiful words that grace the back cover of *Celiac Mom*.

Thank you to bestselling authors and bakers Elana Amsterdam of Elana's Pantry and Peter Reinhart and Denene Wallace for creating wonderful gluten-free recipes and allowing me to share a sample of them in this book.

Thank you to Jill Lake for noticing my concerns about Sydney, being willing to discuss them and suggesting a doctor to see; to Jean Edwards for being a constant and faithful source of support throughout this journey; to Lynn Whitehill for making delicious gluten-free meals and desserts for us, to NorthCross Church for becoming an "allergy-friendly" place of worship; to Megan Ross for inspiring me with your healthy living and inviting Sydney into your life as a mother's helper; to Audrey Butler who created the most amazing birthday cakes ever; to Joanne Schumm and Samantha Hines for always reaching out with love and trying to understand our gluten-free world; to Karen Stewart for providing a safe and welcoming place for Sydney to play and eat, and to the many teachers and friends who were sensitive to Sydney's condition and made an effort to help her feel included and supported.

Thank you to Registered Dietitian Pat Fogarty whose emails and recipes were a lifeline; to the wide network of doctors and healthcare practitioners who provided a diagnosis and much-needed support and healing along the way.

Thank you to the management and staff of Fairhaven Ministries who provided a beautiful, peaceful place for our family to rest, play and learn how to have a gluten-free getaway.

Thank you to friends and the staff at Camp Lurecrest who made it possible for Sydney to experience the fun and joy of camp life; to Polly, Peg and Cassandra who created an unforgettable gluten-free ranch vacation for our family.

Thank you to Lisa Williams Kline and Gilda Morina Syverson for reading drafts of *Celiac Mom*, being willing to talk endlessly about celiac and writing, making suggestions and encouraging me through every step of the publishing process. Thank you to the members of my writing groups who have heard bits and pieces of the book and responded with kind enthusiasm: Jean Beatty, Carolyn Noell, Nancy Lammers, Ruth Ann Grissom, Lisa Williams Kline, Don Carroll, Tootsie O'Hara, Brenda Graham, Suzanne Baldwin Leitner, Dede Mitchell, Allison Elrod, Gilda Morina Syverson and Larry Sorkin.

Thank you to friends and family who made a special effort to understand our unfamiliar eating habits; to my sister who embraced a gluten-free lifestyle along with us and who offered warm encouragement after reading this manuscript; to my sister-in-law Kitty who ordered a supply of gluten-free treats to be delivered to Sydney every month; to my brother-in-law Brian for introducing us to the G-Free Spot on Hilton Head Island and making gluten free Swedish meatballs for Christmas; to Joel's parents who didn't always understand our "food issues" but supported us unconditionally, and to Joel's father Anton who called Sydney "his hero" after reading this manuscript.

This journey would not have been possible (or as much fun) without the wholehearted support of my husband. Thank you, Joel, for always listening and for embracing a gluten-free lifestyle with Sydney and me, even though you've had to give up some of your favorite foods. You have become an awesome shopper over the years, and I'm so glad your golf game has benefitted from this way of eating. I'm grateful for who you are and all you do.

Last, but not least, thank you, especially, to Sydney for allowing me to share your story. I'm blessed to have a daughter who has traveled this road with such strength, vulnerability and grace. Your celiac diagnosis has taught us so much and made our family healthier. Your desire to live a normal and joyful life, your will to succeed and your ability to nourish yourself and others fills me with happiness and pride. Thank you for leading the way. I love you!

Resources: Recipes & Helpful Info

14 Days of Gluten-free Meals

Compiling a list of gluten-free recipes was not the easiest thing for me to do. First off, I'm not a foodie, nor do I like spending loads of time in the kitchen. But these meals kept my family and me fed in the beginning of our gluten-free journey. They have been tested and enjoyed by all of us. And, for the noncooks out there, these meals are easy to make. (Some chicken, other meats and cheeses can be processed with gluten, so be sure you select gluten-free ingredients.)

Johnny Marzetti

This is a meal I grew up eating. While my mom was not a gourmet cook, she had a few meals that we all looked forward to eating. This was one of them. It wasn't hard at all to make it gluten free.

olive oil cooking spray
1 lb ground beef
2 small jars (14 oz) or 1 large jar (24 oz) of GF spaghetti sauce
12 oz of GF noodles (elbow macaroni or fusilli—spiral-shaped—pasta works great) or use 2 boxes (8 oz) of GF spaghetti
1 (8 oz) bag of shredded cheese (cheddar or mozzarella) *or use dairy-free cheese

Preheat oven to 400 degrees. Coat bottom and sides of 9" x 13" baking pan with cooking spray. Brown ground beef in a large pan. Add 2 small jars or 1 large jar of spaghetti sauce to browned meat, simmer on medium low heat, while preparing pasta. Place pasta in boiling water and cook 1-2 minutes less than directions say. Spread cooked pasta in bottom of pan. Pour meat/sauce mix over noodles. Sprinkle bag of shredded cheese on top of meat/sauce mix. Cover baking pan with tin foil. Bake for 30 minutes. Serves 4 to 6 people.

Chicken & Rice

This was another meal that was part of my mom's weekly rotation. Over the years, I changed the white rice to brown and added seasoning to give the chicken more taste.

olive oil cooking spray
6 chicken breasts
2 cups brown rice
24 oz of GF chicken broth (I use Swanson or Pacific, but any GF brands will work as long as you like the taste)
Lawry's or other all-purpose GF seasoning
dash of salt and pepper

Preheat oven to 350 degrees. Coat bottom and sides of 9" x 13" baking dish with cooking spray. Add 2 cups of brown rice. Place chicken breasts on top. Sprinkle liberally with seasoning. Pour 24 oz of chicken broth over chicken. Add salt and pepper. Cover dish with foil. Bake for one hour. Serves 6.

Chicken Pot Pie

This was one of the meals my family most lamented giving up, so I had to come up with a substitute. It is possible to find gluten-free pot pies in the grocery store these days, but often they are a single serving. So, here is an option that fed our family of three and usually gave us leftovers. I like to make a couple of pies at a time, so there's always one in the freezer.

To save time, I buy Wholly Wholesome's Gluten-Free 9" pie crusts, which come 2 in a pack. Then I only have to make the top crust. I usually make 2 pies at a time.

Top Crust (makes enough for 2 crusts, with some leftover)

1 cup white rice flour
½ cup brown rice flour
½ tsp sea salt
1 tsp xanthan gum
2/3 cup butter
4 TB cold water

Mix dry ingredients thoroughly. Add butter and water and mix until a ball of dough forms. Place approximately 1/3 of dough between two pieces of wax paper and roll to desired thickness. Do this a second time, if you are making 2 pies. Place dough (in waxed paper) on cookie sheet in freezer. Move to next step.

Bottom of Pie

2 bags (12 oz) frozen veggies (corn, peas, carrots, green beans)
2 lbs shredded chicken
2 cups chicken broth
Pre-made pie crusts

Preheat oven to 375 degrees. Take 2 pie crust bottoms and fill partway with frozen veggies. I use 1 bag (12 oz) and split it between two pie crusts. Then spread 1 lb of shredded chicken on top of the veggies in each pie. Cover the chicken with the second bag of veggies, splitting it between the two pies. Add 1 cup of chicken broth to each pie. Remove rolled-out crust from freezer. It should be stiff and easy to work with. Place it on top of filled pie crust and cut around the edges with a knife to create a circular crust topping. As the crust warms it will soften and fall into place. Pinch sides together lightly. Use a knife to create slits in the top crust so air will escape. Cover one pie with tin foil and place in freezer for a future meal. Place the other on cookie sheet in oven for 1 hour. Top crust should be slightly golden. Serves 4.

Mom's Modified Meatloaf

Meatloaf was also on my mom's meal rotation. The gluten-filled version was the ONLY meatloaf I would eat as a child. So, it took me a while to attempt modifying it because I just couldn't imagine anything tasting like my mother's recipe. But to my surprise it did. Now I can go back in time whenever I want and taste a bit of home.

    1 lb ground round
    8 oz of GF sausage meat
    1 egg
    salt and pepper to taste
    Glutino GF crackers, 1 handful, crumbled
    dash of milk (I use almond, but any kind is fine)

Preheat oven to 350 degrees. Mix all ingredients together, put in greased loaf pan. Bake for 1 hour. This is my kind of easy! Serves 4 to 6 people.

Sally's Modified Swedish Meatballs/Meatloaf

My husband grew up eating Swedish meatballs every Christmas. It was a treat he always looked forward to. I never dreamed I could replicate his mother's meatballs in a gluten-free fashion, but it was possible. This recipe has more ingredients and steps than most of my meals. But it isn't complicated, and it is worth the effort to bring a smile to my husband's face. Now there are two kinds of meatloaf I will eat.

    1 lb extra lean ground chuck
    1 slice GF bread, broken into bits and soaked in water
    ½ medium baked potato, grated, or 1 large spoon of mashed potatoes
    1 tsp minced onion, dried
    1 tsp salt
    1 tsp sugar
    ½ tsp ground allspice

Preheat oven to 350 degrees. Grease baking pan with sides for meatballs or meatloaf pan for loaf. Combine and mix everything but the meat in a large bowl. Add meat last. For meatloaf, place mixture in loaf pan and bake for 45 minutes to 1 hour. If making meatballs, brown them on pan for 5-10 minutes; turn them over halfway through. When fully cooked, put meatballs in small casserole dish to keep warm. For gravy, mix 1 TB cornstarch in ½ cup water. Mix until smooth. Add salt to taste. Pour water/cornstarch into pan and scrape off bits of meat. Add water/cornstarch/scrapings mixture to casserole dish and heat on stove for 5 minutes. Serves 4 to 6 people.

Homemade Pizza

It took us a while to find a GF pizza crust that didn't taste like cardboard. But when we did, we felt like we'd landed in heaven. We discovered Against the Grain crust when we were in New York, and we bought three of them to take home with us, in case we couldn't find them in North Carolina. Fortunately, this brand is now in many grocery stores. This meal is NOT dairy free. The crust has cheese in it, which is one reason it is so delicious. I no longer eat dairy, but I still remember the joy of that delicious homemade GF pizza.

1 pizza crust (I use Against the Grain, which contains dairy)
1 lb ground, cooked hamburger, GF sausage or several slices of GF pepperoni
1 jar (14 oz) GF pizza sauce
1 bag (8 oz) shredded GF cheese, mozzarella or other

Preheat oven to 400 degrees. On stovetop, cook and break up 1 pound of hamburger or sausage, then set aside. Unwrap pizza crust and place on pizza pan. Spoon out GF pizza sauce onto crust and cover completely. Spread a layer of cooked hamburger/sausage/pepperoni on top of pizza sauce. Sprinkle shredded cheese evenly over the meat. Place pizza in oven on top rack and bake for 10 to 15 minutes, depending on how soft or crunchy you like your pizza. Serves 4.

Hamburger and Macaroni & Cheese

You knew it was coming. This is one of the easiest, cheapest meals around. I used to make the gluten-filled variety for my husband when we were first married. If I could handle the carbs, I'd still be eating it every day.

1 lb ground beef
1 box of GF macaroni and cheese

Brown and crumble ground beef. Set it aside. Follow instructions on box of macaroni and cheese. Then add hamburger to cheesy noodles and stir. If you close your eyes, you can imagine you're eating a cheeseburger. Don't let me start eating this because I can never get enough.

Egg Casserole

This was one of my staples in the early months of going gluten free. Everyone in my family loved it, and it had veggies in it. What could be better? Sometimes I would make up a casserole before Thanksgiving or Christmas and pop it in the oven in the morning. It always impressed my extended family and guests, and they loved it too!

6 large eggs
1 ½ cups milk (I use almond, but have also used regular, skim milk and coconut milk)
1 tsp of mustard powder (this is a key ingredient!)
½ tsp salt
¼ tsp pepper
1 ½ cups of GF shredded cheese
2 slices of GF bread (I use Udi's Multigrain, but any GF bread you like should work)
1 medium yellow squash, thinly sliced
2 cups of broccoli florets

Preheat oven to 350 degrees. Beat eggs, milk, mustard powder, salt and pepper together. Crumble bread into small pieces and add to wet mixture. Slowly add 1 cup of shredded cheese. Then add broccoli florets. Stir until veggies are coated with egg/cheese mixture. Pour entire mixture in a greased pan. (8"x 8" if you like thick and fluffy, 9" x 13" if you like thinner and slightly crispy.) Arrange slices of squash on top of casserole so the sides of each piece are touching. Then sprinkle the last 1/2 cup of cheese on top of the squash. Cover and leave in fridge overnight. Bake for 45 minutes or until the top begins to turn golden brown. Serves 6.

Carolyn's Pot Roast

My friend Carolyn brought me this roast after my mother died. Not to be morbid, but it was so tasty and filling that I made it for several friends who also lost parents. I figured why not pass the love along.

1 cooking bag
Wesson oil
Pam cooking spray
2 ½ to 3 1bs lean chuck roast
2 or 3 large potatoes, quartered or cut in slices
1 dozen small carrots
1 Vidalia onion, large
garlic powder
black pepper
salt
1 cup water

Preheat oven to 325-350 degrees. Brown roast in oil. Spray cooking bag with Pam. Sprinkle roast with garlic powder and black pepper. Put roast inside bag along with carrots, cut-up potatoes, and Vidalia onion. Add salt and pepper to veggies. Add 1 cup of water to bag. Place bag in a large cooking dish or pan. Make sure cooking bag is vented. Cook for 2 to 2½ hours. Check with fork. Roast should be tender. Serves 6.

Chicken and Cheese Tortillas

Every now and then, I get spicy and creative, and this is what I make. It reminds me of the years I lived in Panama, even though my mother never made these.

2 (or more) GF tortillas
1 tsp coconut oil
1 lb cooked chicken, shredded
1 bag (8 oz) of GF shredded cheese, cheddar or mozzarella
1 cup lettuce, chopped
1 tomato, diced
GF salsa
sour cream

Wrap 2 tortillas in a damp paper towel and microwave for 30-45 seconds. Melt coconut oil in large skillet on medium high heat. Place one tortilla in skillet and spread half of it with shredded chicken, lettuce and tomato. Sprinkle cheese on top. Fold tortilla in half and cook until cheese melts. Turn over once, being careful as you flip tortilla to keep it closed. Cook for 1 minute longer. Repeat with second tortilla. Top with salsa and sour cream. 1 or 2 tortillas per person.

Spaghetti

This meal is so easy and obvious I feel guilty adding it to this list of recipes. But my mom used to make it every week, and my family ate it a LOT, especially in the first several years after Sydney's diagnosis. It makes great leftovers! And it is simple to double the recipe.

1 lb ground beef
1 jar (24 oz) of GF spaghetti sauce
2 boxes (8 oz) of spaghetti style rice pasta (I use DeBoles)

Crumble, brown and drain ground beef in a large pot. Mix in spaghetti sauce, cover with lid and simmer for an hour or more. Fill a 3- or 4-quart saucepan with water and bring to a boil. Cook spaghetti for 7 to 9 minutes or follow directions on the box. When the spaghetti is tender, take off the stove immediately and drain. Be aware that GF pasta tends to stick to the pan or dissolve completely, if you let it cook too long. Dish out pasta and add spaghetti sauce. Serves 4 to 6 people.

Hamburger and Corn

My mother's meal rotation included this recipe, except she used Ritz crackers and regular cow's milk. Once again, I surprised myself when I was able to duplicate the flavor. It's an easy, one-dish meal to serve on a cold evening.

4 pieces of bacon (I use Boar's Head microwavable bacon because it's easy)
1 lb ground beef
1 tsp. onion flakes
1 bag (8 oz) of frozen corn
1 cup milk (I use almond)
1 egg
10-12 Glutino GF crackers, crumbled
2 TB butter

Microwave or cook bacon, set aside. Brown the ground beef, stir in onion and crumbled bacon. In a separate bowl, combine corn, milk and egg and mix together with meat. Pour mixture into greased casserole dish (1½ quart). Top with cracker crumbs. Dot mixture with butter. Bake at 350 for 45 minutes. Serves 4.

Homemade Chicken Nuggets or Strips

When all of Sydney's friends were eating chicken nuggets in preschool and Kindergarten, I had to figure this out fast. It was easy but not as easy as zipping through the drive-through.

olive oil cooking spray
1-2 lbs boneless, skinless chicken sliced into nuggets or strips
1 egg, whisked
½ cup milk (I use almond milk)
¾ cup GF breadcrumbs
¼ tsp sea salt
¼ tsp garlic powder
¼ tsp onion powder
dash of pepper

Spray a cookie sheet with olive oil. Combine whisked egg and milk in a small bowl. Combine dry ingredients in a medium bowl. One at a time, dip pieces of chicken into egg and milk mixture. Then drag chicken through dry mixture, being sure to thoroughly coat each piece. Place the coated chicken onto the cookie sheet. Bake at 350 degrees for 15 minutes. Serves 4.

Chicken Fried Rice

I love fried rice and miss the good old days when my husband and I could indulge in Chinese takeout. We used to eat it every New Year's Eve. This is not a difficult dish to prepare, but I rarely make it, probably because it requires thinking ahead. When it comes to meals, that's not my strong suit. But if you're a better food planner than I am, and you have rice and chicken already made and stored in the fridge, you won't have a problem. Fried rice takes only a few minutes to prepare, and everyone always wants seconds!

6 cups brown or white rice, cooked and chilled
1 lb boneless, skinless, cooked chicken, sliced into thin pieces
1 cup veggies (frozen sweet peas and carrots)
2 TB olive oil
½ tsp garlic
½ tsp dried onion flakes
2 eggs, beaten
3 TB GF soy sauce

Preheat large frying pan over medium heat. Add 1 TB oil and stir in garlic and onion. Reduce heat to medium and add eggs. Scramble eggs, breaking into small pieces. Add chicken and stir until heated. Remove chicken and egg from pan and set aside.

Add second TB of oil to pan and turn heat up to medium. Add rice and cook for 2 minutes, until toasted. Add chicken, eggs, veggies and soy sauce. Cook for 1-2 more minutes, until frozen veggies are steamed. Serve hot and enjoy! Serves 4 to 6.

Recipes from the Professionals

There are tons of gluten-free websites and cookbooks out there these days. Here are sample recipes from some of my favorite "real" cooks.

Elana's Pantry (https://elanaspantry.com/)

Elana's Pantry is one of my favorite go-to websites. Elana is not only a fabulous cook, but she has celiac disease herself. So, everything she makes is gluten free. Her site is a treasure trove of delicious recipes, and they are well organized. She even categorizes them for different diets, so if you have allergies to ingredients like eggs or dairy, you can easily find what you need. Here's a sample, just to give you a taste (pun intended) of what she offers. These sugar cookies make holiday baking possible for us because everyone knows decorating cookies is a requirement at Christmas!

Paleo Sugar Cookies from Elana's Pantry

    3 cups blanched almond flour (not almond meal)
    ½ tsp celtic sea salt
    ¼ tsp baking soda
    1 pinch ground nutmeg
    ½ cup coconut oil, melted
    ¼ cup honey
    1 TB orange zest

In a large bowl, combine almond flour, salt, baking soda and nutmeg. In a small bowl, mix together coconut oil, honey and orange zest. Mix wet ingredients into dry. Separate dough into 2 balls and place each on a piece of parchment paper. Cover each ball of dough with another piece of parchment paper and roll out ¼ inch thick. Place in freezer for 30 minutes. Use heart-shaped [or Christmas] cookie cutters to cut out cookies. Bake at 350°F for 5 to 7 minutes. Cool and serve. Makes 32 cookies.

Check out Elana's cookbooks too. *Paleo Cooking from Elana's Pantry, Gluten-Free Cupcakes* and *The Gluten-Free, Almond Flour Cookbook.*

The Joy of Gluten-Free, Sugar-Free Baking by Peter Reinhart & Denene Wallace (https://www.amazon.com/Joy-Gluten-Free-Sugar-Free-Baking-Solutions-ebook/dp/B008C84EPO)

I received this cookbook as a gift from my sister a few years after Sydney was diagnosed. What a great collection of breads, pizzas, crackers, muffins, cookies, cakes and more. I was delighted to find that I could make all these things gluten free *and* sugar free! These recipes are two of my favorites from the book. I have to hold myself back from eating an entire loaf of bread at once, and after feeding my family pancakes for breakfast, there are never any leftovers.

Toasting Bread

Makes 1 large loaf (10-12 slices), or 4 to 6 mini loaves

2 cups (8 oz / 227 g) brown or golden flaxseed meal
2 cups (8 oz / 227 g) pecan flour
¼ cup (1.15 oz / 32 g) sesame seeds
¼ cup (1.4 oz / 40 g) whole flaxseeds (optional)
4 tsp baking powder
1 tsp xanthan gum
½ tsp salt
1½ cups (12 oz / 340 g) unsweetened soy milk or other milk
8 egg whites (10 oz / 283 g)
¼ to ½ tsp liquid stevia (optional)

Preheat the oven to 375 degrees F (191 degrees C). Line the bottom of a 4½ x 8-inch loaf pan with parchment paper, then mist the pan with spray oil. (If making mini loaves, forgo the parchment paper and simply coat the pans generously with spray oil.)

In a medium bowl, combine the flaxseed meal, pecan flour, sesame seeds, flaxseeds, baking powder, xanthan gum and salt and whisk until well mixed. In a large bowl, whisk the milk, egg whites and liquid stevia together until thoroughly blended. Add the flour mixture and stir vigorously with a large spoon for about 2 minutes to make a thick, sticky, slightly aerated batter.

Pour the mixture into the prepared pan or pans, filling them to about ½ inch from the top. For a large loaf, bake for 45 minutes, then rotate and bake for 25 to 30 minutes. The bread is fully cooked when golden brown and springy when pressed in the center.

Transfer to a wire rack and let cool for at least 5 minutes. Before turning out the loaf, run an icing spatula or thin knife around the edges to loosen the bread from the sides. Cool for at least 15 more minutes before slicing. Store the bread in the refrigerator.

Everyday Pancakes

Makes 8 to 10 four- to six-inch pancakes

1 cup (4 oz / 113 g) hazelnut flour
1 cup (4 oz / 113 g) almond flour
¼ cup Stevia Extract in the Raw, or 2 TB New Roots Stevia Sugar
1 tsp baking powder
¼ tsp salt
1 egg (1.75 oz / 50 g)
½ cup (4 oz / 113 g) unsweetened soy milk or other milk
¼ cup (2 oz / 57 g) water
1 tsp vanilla extract (optional)

In a medium bowl, combine the hazelnut flour, almond flour, sweetener, baking powder and salt and whisk until well mixed. In a large bowl, whisk the egg, milk, water and vanilla together until thoroughly blended. Add the flour mixture and stir with a large spoon or whisk just until all of the ingredients are evenly blended into a loose, pourable batter.

Heat a nonstick griddle or skillet over medium heat. When a few drops of water splashed on the surface sizzle and evaporate quickly, the pan is hot enough for cooking pancakes. Mist the pan with spray oil or put about 1 teaspoon of butter or margarine on the pan and swirl to coat the surface.

Portion pancakes onto the pan, using about ¼ cup of batter per pancake and leaving a bit of space between them. The batter should sizzle when it hits the pan. Lower the heat to medium-low and cook the first side for about 4 minutes, until the bottom is golden brown, and the top begins to dry out. Flip pancakes over and cook the second side for 3 to 4 minutes, until the center is springy when pressed. Serve hot.

Helpful People, Podcasts, Websites and Products

An assortment of people, podcasts, websites and products that have helped us on our gluten-free journey.

BeyondCeliac.org
Website: https://www.beyondceliac.org/

The Celiac Project Podcast
Website: https//www.celiacproject.com/the-podcast

The Healthy Celiac Podcast
Website: https://www.belindawhelan.com/thehealthyceliacpodcast

A Canadian Celiac Podcast
Website: https://acanadianceliacpodcast.libsyn.com/

Pat Fogarty, Registered Dietitian Nutritionist
patfogartyrdn@gmail.com

Deleon Best
Best Acupuncture
Website: https://bestacupuncture.com/

Akiba Green
Lake Norman Health and Wellness
Website: https://www.drakibagreen.com/

Nima Partners: a portable gluten tester.
Website: https://nimapartners.com/
Nima uses antibody-based chemistry to test samples of food for proteins found in gluten. A handy tool to have when you're going out to eat and you're not sure you trust the restaurant or the chef.

Shopping List *

*Companies constantly change and update their ingredients, so always check labels to make sure the product is gluten free.

Gluten-free Meats

Fresh meat that is unseasoned and not marinated should be gluten free. But if you are not sure, it is always a good idea to ask.

Chicken
  Boar's Head deli meats (all varieties)
  D&W deli meats (most varieties, check label, it will say)
  Jennie-O chicken (most varieties)
  Perdue – ground chicken, shortcuts, individual frozen breasts, tender loins & wings
  Swanson – premium chunk white chicken (canned)

Turkey
  Butterball (most varieties)
  Boar's head
  Healthy Choice (golden, honey roasted)
  Jennie-O
  Perdue
  Wellshire Farms

Gluten-free Snacks

  any raw fruit or vegetables without seasoning or sauce
  microwave popcorn – Pop Secret, Jolly Time, Newman's Own
  Fritos Corn Chips
  nuts – Planters, Blue Diamond
  Tostitos Crispy Round Tortilla Chips & other tortilla/corn chips
  Lays & Baked Lays Potato Chips
  Cracker Jacks – Original Flavor
  Cheetos

Yoplait Yogurt
EnviroKidz GF crispy rice bars
Welch's Fruit Snacks

Gluten-free Odds & Ends

Udi's bread and bagels
Against the Grain Pizza Crust
Peanut butter – Jiff, Skippy
Jelly – most varieties, Smuckers, Welch's
Ore-Ida French Fries and Tater Tots
Ken's salad dressings (most varieties)
Amy's frozen GF macaroni & cheese
Annie's (in a box) GF macaroni & cheese
Corn tortillas
Progresso Soups
  Chicken Rice with Vegetables
  Creamy Mushroom
  Chicken Corn Chowder
Pacific Foods
  Broths and stocks
Swanson
  Broths and stocks
Frozen veggies with no sauce
  Del Monte
  Birds Eye
  Green Giant
Bush's Best BBQ baked beans, original baked, honey baked, homestyle baked & others
Van's GF Frozen Waffles

Ice Cream
  So Delicious
  Breyers (vanilla, chocolate, strawberry)
  Edy's (vanilla, butter pecan & other flavors)

Gluten-free Candy

Candy companies often change suppliers and ingredients, so be sure to double-check these before buying.

M&Ms (plain & peanut)
Starbursts
Hershey's kisses
SweetTarts
Baby Ruth
Butterfinger
3 Musketeers
Starburst Jelly Beans
Jelly Belly Jelly Beans
Tootsie Rolls
Dum Dum pops

Eating Out

These are gluten-free items our family has enjoyed from fast-food restaurants and eating establishments. But many of these places do NOT have dedicated gluten-free preparation areas, so proceed with caution. Make it a habit to discuss your condition with the waitstaff, restaurant manager and/or chef before ordering. Depending on your level of sensitivity, food items are not always safe for those with celiac disease. Here are some of our favorites.

Wendy's – chili, baked potatoes, Caesar salad, Frosty's (vanilla & original flavor)

Chick Fil-A – French fries, grilled chicken with no bun and grilled nuggets, fruit cup

Five Guys – burgers in lettuce wrap or bowl, French fries, peanuts

Dairy Queen – soft serve ice cream (vanilla & chocolate)

Panera Bread – some salads (with no croutons or bread)

Boston Market – roasted turkey and gravy, chicken, steamed veggies, mashed potatoes

Burtons Grill & Bar – hamburgers with GF buns, sweet potato fries

Outback Steak House – steak, baked potatoes

Mellow Mushroom – GF pizza, salads (with no croutons or bread)

P.F. Chang's – beef with broccoli, fried rice (both from GF menu)

Chipotle – bowl with chicken, rice, beans and queso

CAVA – salad bowl with grilled chicken and grilled veggies

Bad Daddy's – hamburgers, salads (with no croutons or bread)

Brixx Pizza – GF pizza, salads (with no croutons or bread)

Carrabba's – grilled chicken, broccoli, mashed potatoes

Snooze – GF blueberry pancakes, eggs and bacon

About the Author

Ann Campanella is a former magazine and newspaper editor. She is the author of *Motherhood: Lost and Found*, an award-winning memoir, and four collections of poems. Her work has appeared in newspapers, magazines, literary journals and online sites across the country and around the world, and she has discussed her writing on numerous podcasts. In 2018, Ann was recognized by her hometown newspaper as one of the Most Influential Women in her community. She is a manager and director of AlzAuthors.com, a website that represents hundreds of books about Alzheimer's and dementia. Ann has a degree in English Literature from Davidson College and lives on a small farm with her family and animals in North Carolina. For more information about the author and her books, visit AnnCampanella.com.

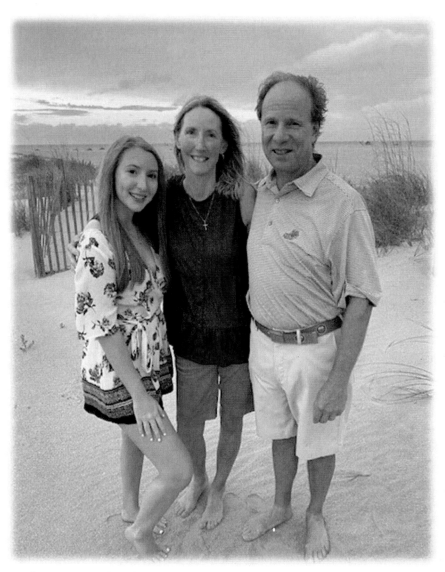

Sydney, Ann and Joel Campanella, June 2020.

THE BRIDGE

A medium that transports
story from inspiration to creation.
Our desire is that authors and readers
will be affirmed through
creativity and the written word.

More books by Ann Campanella

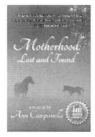 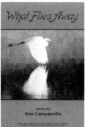 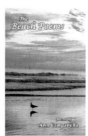

Motherhood: Lost and Found
This award-winning memoir takes the reader on a journey where horses, Alzheimer's disease and infertility intersect, connecting the reader to the heartbeat and resilience of the human spirit. Named "One of the Best Alzheimer's Books of All-Time" by Book Authority. Available in softcover, Kindle and audiobook.

What Flies Away
This collection of poems tells the story of the author's mother's descent into Alzheimer's, her father's sudden death and the miracle of her daughter's birth. Ann Campanella received the Poet Laureate Award twice for two poems, "The Chase" and "How to Grieve," both of which are included in this volume of poetry. Available in softcover and Kindle.

The Beach Poems
This collection of poetry was inspired by Anne Morrow Lindbergh's *Gift from the Sea*. After caring for a loved one who had Alzheimer's for 14 years, Ann Campanella went on a series of retreats at the beach. These retreats inspired memories and nourished her soul, ultimately carrying the author through grief to a place of joy. Available in softcover.

Order from Amazon or through your local bookstore.
For more information,
visit www.thebridgebooks.com.

Made in United States
North Haven, CT
24 February 2025

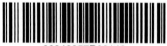

66242957R00148